The Dr. Gundry's Diet Cookbook

80+ Gut-Friendly Recipes Inspired by Dr. Steven Gundry's Teachings to Help Restore Health, Lose Weight, and Heal Your Microbiome

---

Sonia Jones

Copyright © 2025 Sonia Jones
All rights reserved.

No part of this book may be reproduced, distributed, or transmitted in any form or by any means, including photocopying, recording, or other electronic or mechanical methods, without the prior written permission of the author, except in the case of brief quotations used in reviews or critical analyses.

Disclaimer

This book is inspired by the teachings of Dr. Steven Gundry but is not affiliated with or endorsed by Dr. Gundry or his organization. The recipes and recommendations provided are for informational purposes only and should not be considered a substitute for professional medical advice, diagnosis, or treatment.

Always consult a qualified healthcare provider or nutritionist before making significant changes to your diet, especially if you have a medical condition, are pregnant, or are taking medication. The author and publisher are not responsible for any adverse effects, outcomes, or consequences resulting from the use or application of the information provided in this book.

About the Author

Dr. Steven R. Gundry, MD, is a famous cardiac surgeon, medical researcher, and New York Times bestselling author who has transformed the subject of nutrition and health. Dr. Gundry has become a leading champion for gut health and its impact on overall well-being, thanks to decades of medical experience, breakthrough research, and an uncompromising commitment to improving health outcomes.

Dr. Gundry received his medical degree from the Medical College of Georgia and completed his surgical residency at the University of Michigan. He went on to receive further training in cardiothoracic surgery at the reputed National Institutes of Health (NIH). As one of the most skilled cardiac surgeons of his time, Dr. Gundry played a key role in establishing new surgical techniques, including some life-saving operations that have subsequently become industry standards.

Throughout his successful medical career, Dr. Gundry performed thousands of difficult heart procedures and was the Head of Cardiothoracic Surgery at Loma Linda University Medical Center. His pioneering work garnered him worldwide recognition, including awards for achieving exceptional survival rates in high-risk patients.

In the late 1990s, Dr. Gundry had a watershed moment that would change his career. He met a patient who had successfully corrected major cardiac disease with an unorthodox nutritional regimen. Inspired by this, Dr. Gundry began researching the link between nutrition, gut wellness, and chronic diseases.

This path led to the establishment of the International Heart & Lung Institute, and then the Center for Restorative Medicine, where Dr. Gundry specialized in treating patients with chronic illnesses using dietary treatments. His research revealed that lectins, which are plant-based proteins, play an important role in generating inflammation and autoimmune reactions. This revelation created the groundwork for his "Plant Paradox" program, a new eating strategy that prioritizes intestinal health, decreases inflammation, and promotes overall well-being.

Dr. Gundry has written several best-selling books that turn his extensive study into practical guidance for daily people. His most significant works include:

The Plant Paradox: The Hidden Risks in "Healthy" Foods That Cause Disease and Weight Gain
The Longevity Paradox: How to Die Young in a Ripe Old Age
The Energy Paradox: What to Do When Your Get-Up-and-Go Is Gone

These books have inspired millions to reconsider their diets and adopt a lifestyle that promotes long-term health. His writing blends cutting-edge science and practical ideas, making difficult medical topics understandable to a broad readership.

Dr. Gundry's research highlights the significance of the gut flora in supporting general health. He highlights that many chronic conditions, such as autoimmune disorders, obesity, and heart disease, can be reduced or even reversed by improving gut health. In his dietary advice, he argues for reducing inflammatory foods, embracing nutrient-dense ingredients, and combining prebiotics and probiotics to nurture the microbiota.

To broaden the accessibility of his teachings, Dr. Gundry launched Gundry MD, a firm dedicated to delivering high-quality supplements, meals, and resources that promote gut health and longevity. Gundry MD's product line is based on his decades of clinical experience and scientific study, providing practical answers for anyone looking to better their health.

Preface

Welcome to *The Dr. Gundry's Diet Cookbook: 80+ Gut-Friendly Recipes Inspired by Dr. Steven Gundry's Teachings to Help Restore Health, Lose Weight, and Heal Your Microbiome*. This book is a labor of love, inspired by the groundbreaking principles of Dr. Steven R. Gundry, MD—a pioneer in nutritional science and an advocate for the transformative power of gut health.

Over the past few decades, Dr. Gundry's research and teachings have revolutionized how we approach food, shedding light on the hidden dangers in some of the most commonly consumed "healthy" foods and offering actionable solutions to support the body's natural ability to heal. His work has empowered millions to take charge of their health, and I am honored to present this cookbook as a practical companion for anyone who wants to embrace his wisdom in their daily lives.

This book is not just a collection of recipes; it's an invitation to transform your relationship with food. Each recipe has been carefully crafted to align with Dr. Gundry's dietary principles, focusing on eliminating harmful lectins, reducing inflammation, and restoring the delicate balance of your gut microbiome. These recipes prove that eating for health doesn't mean sacrificing flavor or joy. From hearty breakfasts to satisfying dinners and even guilt-free desserts, this cookbook provides a variety of options that are as delicious as they are nourishing.

You'll also find tips and insights throughout the book to help you understand the science behind Dr. Gundry's approach. Whether you're new to his teachings or a longtime follower, these recipes will guide you toward better health, improved energy, and sustainable weight loss.

As someone who has personally experienced the transformative power of Dr. Gundry's principles, I can attest to the life-changing benefits of this way of eating. By focusing on foods that truly nourish the body, I've discovered a new level of vitality and wellness that I didn't think was possible. It is my hope that this cookbook will serve as a resource and inspiration for you to embark on your own journey to optimal health.

Thank you for choosing this book as a part of your health and wellness journey. May it be a source of knowledge, encouragement, and delicious meals that bring you closer to your goals.

To your health and happiness,
Sonia Jones

Introduction

My Healing Story

Six years ago, I was forced to undergo a major life shift after being diagnosed with a non-specific (meaning it affected multiple organs) autoimmune disease and fibromyalgia. My healing journey was difficult in the early years. I spent three months languishing in a hospital bed, coping with my disease and terrible arthritis. I dropped nearly 33 pounds (15 kg); hives and bruises covered my entire body from head to toe; and I experienced brain fog, hair loss, and great weariness. There were numerous days when I couldn't muster enough energy to get out of bed.

Consider your gut to be a garden that can only bloom in healthy soil. Healthy soil necessitates healthy meals and nutrients, which will enable the "good guys" to thrive. By giving my body all-natural, easily digestible wholefoods, I enabled it to repair on a fundamental level.

During my stay in the hospital, I was given a variety of medications, ranging from immunosuppressants and antibiotics to steroids, anticancer treatments, and anti-inflammatories. All of this was done to reduce inflammation in my body. The main issue was that the medications made me feel worse, with Alfred Hitchcock-like side effects! I felt sick, fatigued, hazy, and fuzzy. During my nutrition studies, I believed that pharmaceutical medications simply treated symptoms of diseases. Most days, when I awoke from sporadic and disrupted sleep, I felt like a forty-year-old trapped in an eighty-year-old woman's body, like Benjamin Button reversed. I was bent double, unable to get out of bed, and my lovely thick hair was falling out in clumps on my pillow.

As I lay there, I pondered whether my illness was diet-related, and if I repaired my stomach and allowed my system to recuperate, I'd be able to regain my energy and health. I made a conscious commitment to research health and sickness to understand the root cause of my ailment and find natural healing methods. Thus began the process of controlling my own medical destiny. When I initially got sick, I was on an extremely tight diet since my body responded to everything I ate, and I was accumulating allergies and intolerances. To improve digestion and nutrient absorption, I started consuming mostly liquid foods. This procedure of carefully mending my gut lining took around four weeks, but it allowed my digestive system to improve and recuperate.

When my gut felt better and I was in less discomfort, I began taking probiotics and consuming probiotic-rich foods to repair my gut and restore my gut microflora (my "good" bacteria). When my gut started to recover, I began consuming nutrient-dense foods. My health improved significantly as I ingested and absorbed more nutrients.

I still have an autoimmune disease. My arthritic symptoms flare up on rainy or cold days, but I now know how to control them, and they no longer interfere with my life as much as they formerly did. I live an energetic, healthy, and full life, and the gastrointestinal protocol I followed, as well as the food plan I'm currently on, have improved my quality of life. I'm no longer on any prescription drugs, and I'm 90% recovered. It would be untrue to suggest that I would ever feel completely healthy, but accepting my 90% and focusing on enjoying every moment of life has been a significant part of my healing process.

Healing my gut was an important part of restoring my health and vitality, and I want to share what I've learned with you so you, too, can heal your gut and reclaim your life.

Chapter 1

The Importance of Your Gut

INSIDE YOUR GUT

To begin my journey of naturally curing the symptoms of my autoimmune condition, I had to conduct extensive research on the stomach and how it influences health. Your gut is more than simply your stomach or waistline; it is the entryway to the health of your brain and immune system. Hippocrates, the ancient Greek physician, stated two thousand years ago that "all disease begins in the gut." It appears that today more than ever, we should heed this advise and look at the source of many of our health problems: the gut.

Hippocrates is regarded as the father of medicine, yet modern medicine has diverged significantly from his ideas, focusing on cures rather than causes. While Hippocrates' message has been tragically disregarded for millennia, recent research is pointing to the reality and profundity of his simple premise. Indeed, many researchers believe that sustaining gut health and restoring gut barrier integrity will be among the most important goals of medicine in the twenty-first century.

GUT FLORA

Did you know that your body is home to over 100 trillion living organisms? Although you can't see it, your body is covered in bacteria. They outnumber your cells ten-to-one. They live everywhere, including your hair, skin, nose, and mouth! The gut contains the highest concentration of these microscopic bacteria.

Microflora are living creatures that form a complex, interrelated, and interdependent connection within your gut. The microflora is a complex and diverse set of microorganisms that live in your digestive tract. These organisms, often known as gut flora, are most readily classified as "good bacteria" or "bad bacteria."

Although "good" or "friendly" bacteria

carry out a wide range of functions in your body, they frequently work to maintain gut balance by removing some of the toxic byproducts of digestion; inhibit the growth of pathogenic bacteria; regulate metabolism; lower harmful substances like toxins and carcinogens; extract and absorb energy, nutrients, and fatty acids from food; recycle hormones; strengthen the immune system; and communicate with your brain.

There are numerous, interrelated, and interdependent relationships between the different kinds of microorganisms in your gut.

"Bad bacteria" are germs that can cause sickness in the body by infecting cells and increasing the risk of cancer. Research suggests that pathogenic bacteria in mice might cause obesity, metabolic damage, and insulin resistance.

Researchers are learning more and more about the vital role of gut flora in overall health. Dysregulation of gut flora has been related to a variety of disorders, including autism and depression, as well as autoimmune conditions like Hashimoto's thyroiditis, inflammatory bowel disease (IBD), and type 1 diabetes.

A healthy gut flora balance consists of roughly 85% beneficial bacteria and 15% harmful bacteria. However, our modern diet, which is high in sugar, carbs, preservatives, and additives, is ideal for the growth of harmful bacteria, which will soon deplete your beneficial gut flora.

Other sources of this imbalance include modern antibiotics and drinking tap water, which contains chemicals like fluoride and chlorine, both of which kill healthy bacteria. If you experience acne, low energy, digestive issues, or low immunity, you may have a gut-flora imbalance that requires treatment.

Senior scientists at the American Gut Project in Colorado are currently analyzing feces samples from people all over the world in order to correlate their specific ecological community of gut microbes (known as the microbiome or microbiota) with various diseases. The human microbiome is thought to play a role in autoimmune disorders such as diabetes, rheumatoid arthritis, muscular dystrophy, multiple sclerosis, and fibromyalgia.

CANDIDA AND THE GUT

An imbalance in your gut flora can cause an overgrowth of Candida (Candida albicans), a fungus that naturally exists in the human body and aids digestion and nutrition absorption. Good bacteria regulate candida levels when they become imbalanced. If your microflora is uneven, candida can become destructive, tearing down the gut wall and seeping into the bloodstream, releasing toxic by-products into your body and causing a slew of debilitating symptoms. If you have an autoimmune condition, there is a good risk that your gut microflora is out of balance, resulting in an overgrowth of yeast.

Coconut oil is a heart-healthy saturated fat that regulates cholesterol and boosts immunological function. Coconut oil includes lauric acid, an effective antiviral, antibacterial, and antifungal agent that is easily digested and absorbed. It promotes detoxification, digestion, and nutritional absorption. The best coconut oil to buy is cold or expeller-pressed, unrefined. It is the ideal oil for cooking due to its high smoke point.

TEN COMMON CANDIDA SYMPTOMS

- Chronic weariness, lethargy, and brain fog.
- Muscle and joint discomfort and bromyalgia
- Fungal diseases of the skin and nails, such as athlete's foot or toenail fungus
- Oral and vaginal thrush, urinary tract infections, rectal or vaginal itching.
- Irritable bowel syndrome (IBS) includes digestive disorders, such as bloating, gas, constipation, or diarrhoea, as well as new sensitivities to commonly consumed foods
- Autoimmune illnesses include Hashimoto's thyroiditis, rheumatoid arthritis, ulcerative colitis, lupus, psoriasis, scleroderma, and multiple sclerosis.
- inability to concentrate, confusion, poor memory, loss of focus, attention deficit hyperactivity disorder (ADHD), and headaches
- Skin and allergy issues include sinusitis, itching, hay fever, eczema, psoriasis, hives, rashes, and recurring colds or tonsillitis.
- Mood fluctuations, anxiety or depression, impatience, and heart palpitations
- Alcohol intolerance, sensitivity to chemicals and fragrances, appetites for sugar and refined carbohydrates, and heightened vulnerability to drug adverse effects.

SIMPLE YEAST TEST

Here is a simple test you may use to determine whether yeast has overgrown in your body. It takes 15 minutes and only requires a glass of water and a

sample of your own saliva.
This is how you do it:

Within 30 minutes of awakening, fill a glass with water and spit into it. Make sure you do it before you rinse, spit, or consume anything.

Wait 15 minutes, then check your results:

NORMAL: Your saliva floats at the surface.

HIGH LEVELS OF YEAST: The glass becomes foggy, and your saliva settles to the bottom like sediment. If your saliva floats but has little threads dropping down into the water, resembling a jellyfish, or if you notice particles in the water, you may have too much yeast in your system.

If you're concerned about your yeast levels, see your local integrative medical practitioner. They can take swabs, blood, stool, or urine samples to check for yeast overgrowth.

REBALANCING YOUR YEAST LEVELS

Candida and bad bacteria live on sugar, thus it's critical to avoid sweets for a period of time to eliminate the nasty bacteria in your gut. Any item that quickly breaks down into sugar - white bread, white rice - as well as a diet strong in fruit or carbohydrates, such as spaghetti and even oats, can provide a feast for nasty bacteria. Avoiding these foods as much as possible over a period of time will starve harmful bacteria and keep them from outnumbering good bacteria.

Increasing your intake of dietary fiber, anti-inflammatory good fats like extra virgin olive oil, flaxseed (linseed) oil, cold-pressed extra virgin coconut oil, and avocados, as well as antioxidant-rich foods, will aid in the elimination and destruction of harmful bacteria.

Garlic is an especially effective natural antiseptic. It has been demonstrated to be effective against 24 of the 26 strains of candida. It eliminates harmful germs while increasing beneficial bacteria. Garlic was one of my most powerful partners as I worked to heal my gut.

Fiber-rich foods, such as nuts and seeds, as well as an abundance of fresh vegetables, including leafy greens, will eliminate candida and other yeasts from your system while also alkalizing the magical world inside, encouraging a healthy gut-flora balance. According to University of Illinois research, consuming dietary fiber can improve gut bacteria health and shift the microbiome towards more beneficial bacteria. Fiber is essential for our gut environment and keeps it in balance.

Supplements including oil of oregano, black walnut, burdock root, goldenseal, olive leaf extract, grapefruit seed extract, and pau d'arco are effective natural remedies for eliminating candida and yeast. When taking supplements, it's vital to introduce them gradually and one at a time to avoid overwhelming your body. Always follow your healthcare practitioner's dose recommendations. The golden rule is to avoid starting any anti-candida program too quickly.

Garlic is a highly effective natural antiseptic. It has been demonstrated to be effective against 24 out of 26 Candida strains. It eliminates harmful germs while promoting beneficial bacteria.

HEALING AND MAINTAINING A HEALTHY GUT BARRIER

It's important to understand your internal flora, and there are tests available to determine the exact quantities of specific bacteria in your stomach. Gut flora, however, is only one aspect of the gut-health equation. Healing and maintaining a healthy intestinal barrier is another critical aspect.

The gut barrier extends from your mouth to your anus, and its principal function, aside from delivering and discarding food and fluids, is to keep external, undesired substances from entering the body. To function properly, the intestinal barrier must be strong and healthy. Unfortunately, due to poor modern lifestyles, gut permeability or "leaky gut" is becoming a widespread condition. This includes the breakdown of intestinal walls, resulting in "holes" that allow big protein molecules to escape into the body. The immune system attacks these proteins as invaders because they are not normally found outside the gut. This behaviour is thought to be a leading cause of autoimmune diseases. I discovered that as soon as I began mending my gut lining, my problems subsided.

Although mainstream medicine formerly dismissed this theory, many medical experts and researchers are now acknowledging that the integrity of the intestinal barrier is critical in avoiding and treating a variety of disorders.

A very essential element to remember on your own healing journey is that mending the gut requires a dual focus: increasing the balance of healthy bacteria in the gut and healing the intestinal walls to reduce intestinal permeability. By doing so, you allow your stomach to do all of the processes necessary to manage your entire body without leaking undesirable toxic compounds into the bloodstream, lowering your risk of acquiring numerous ailments.

THE GUT AND IMMUNE SYSTEM CONNECTION

All of your body's systems work together to maintain optimal health, so when one is out of balance, it can cause difficulties in other areas of your body, resulting in a cascade of chronic health complications. This is especially true for the gut and its effect on immunological health. Your intestinal health and immune system are intricately related. Did you know that 70-80% of your immunological tissue is found in your digestive system? The gut is frequently the primary entry site for pathogens (bad bacteria and viruses that can cause disease); so, your gut immune system must be flourishing and healthy in order for you to avoid illness. I was motivated to mend my intestines since I knew it would relieve my symptoms.

The immune system is your first line of defense. A healthy balance of beneficial bacteria in the gut is essential for the immune system to function properly and defend against infections.

The digestive system is made up of cells, proteins, tissues, and organs that work together in a complicated manner to protect the body from harmful germs, infectious diseases, and toxins. In reality, the gut mucosa, which forms the intestinal barrier, interacts with the body's biggest population of immune cells, known as gastrointestinal immune cells. These arise from the immune system's lymphoid branch and include lymphocyte cells that combat dangerous invaders. These lymphatic cells generate Peyer's patches, which protect the small intestine's mucous membranes against infection. They accomplish this by releasing specialized white blood cells (lymphocytes) known as T-cells and B-cells to protect the inside of the digestive tract from infection and repair the damage caused by harmful bacteria to the intestinal walls.

The intestinal barrier also supports friendly gut bacteria, which are essential for overall immunity. These guys serve as formidable warriors for the immune system and dependable partners for immune cells, assisting them in increasing their "natural killer" effectiveness and strengthening their general defense of the intestinal walls to prevent pathogens and diseases from entering the bloodstream. This is why keeping a healthy balance of beneficial bacteria in the gut is critical. Without them, your immune system is unable to function properly and is basically defenceless.

Slippery elm has been utilized for food and medicine in various herbal traditions, including Native American, Ayurvedic, traditional Chinese, and Western medicine. It is highly nutritious and can be consumed as a meal.

HOW TO MAKE SLIPPERY ELM PORRIDGE

In a blender, combine 1-2 tablespoons slippery elm inner bark powder, 1/4 teaspoon powdered stevia, 1/2 teaspoon vanilla essence, 1/4 teaspoon cinnamon, and 1 cup (9 oz/250 ml) almond milk. Blend until smooth. Pour the mixture into a small saucepan and cook over low heat, stirring regularly, until it thickens to the consistency of soft porridge. Remove from the heat, transfer to a bowl, and eat immediately.

HEALING A LEAKY GUT

When the gut's defensive activities are impaired, a number of ailments can develop. As previously noted, intestinal permeability, often known as 'leaky gut', leads the immune system to overreact to things like gluten, harmful bacteria, and undigested foods that have gone through these permeable holes in the gut lining. One of the earliest signs of leaky gut is an increase in dietary intolerances. If left untreated, this might cause immunological irregularities, autoimmune diseases, and other health problems. IBD, arthritis, eczema, psoriasis, depression, migraine headaches, muscle pain, fibromyalgia, chronic tiredness, colitis, type 1 diabetes, Graves' disease, thyroiditis, multiple sclerosis, lupus, scleroderma, Crohn's disease, and Addison's disease are a few examples.

If you suspect you have a leaky gut, nourishing slippery elm porridge will help you seal the stomach lining. The herb slippery elm has been demonstrated to neutralize acidity and function as a soothing demulcent by covering the membrane surface and preserving mucous membranes throughout the digestive tract. Slippery elm porridge effectively soothes inflamed intestines by isolating the acidic environment and stimulating tissue regeneration. It relieves constipation without causing bloating. Slippery elm has been utilized for food and medicine in various herbal traditions, including Native American, Ayurvedic, traditional Chinese, and Western medicine. This porridge is highly nutritious and can be enjoyed as a meal.

If your leaky gut is extremely difficult,

eat it three times a day for three days to aid in gut repair, then return to eating it as a meal replacement as needed. For a small drink, combine 1 teaspoon slippery elm powder with 1/2 cup (4 fl oz/125 ml) warm water and consume 30 minutes before meals.

Only in recent years have scientists come to recognize the critical importance of the linkages between nutrition, gut flora, and the immune system. Scientific research now indicates that the sorts of food you consume directly influence the amounts of particular bacteria in your gut. Changing your food can alter the microorganisms in your body, either increasing or weakening your immune system. The current research concludes that a strong immune system is the outcome of a diet that promotes healthy gut function - one that emphasizes whole, unprocessed foods and aids in the repopulation of the gut with beneficial bacteria.

THE GUT AND BRAIN CONNECTION

The gut is not only closely linked to your immune system; the health of your digestive system has a direct impact on the functioning of your brain. The gut-brain axis demonstrates the interdependence of these two parts of the body. In fact, your body has two nervous systems: the central nervous system, which includes your brain and spinal cord, and the enteric nervous system, which is the intrinsic neural system of your digestive tract.

During fetal development, your two nervous systems are produced simultaneously and are made up of identical components that are joined by the vagus nerve. This is the tenth cranial nerve, which extends from the brain stem to your abdomen and serves as the principal conduit for gut microbes to communicate with your brain. Understanding the vagus nerve completely challenges the notion that the brain controls the rest of your body. Rather, it demonstrates that your stomach is mainly in control. In reality, your gut transmits significantly more information to your brain than the other way around!

Neurons exist in both the brain and the gut. This includes neurons that create neurotransmitters like serotonin. Serotonin is the neurotransmitter responsible for emotions of well-being and happiness, and it is more concentrated in the gut rather than the brain. When my autoimmune condition initially flared up, I experienced severe anxiety and depression. This was due to a combination of steroid use and anxiety, as well as a lack of healthy gut microbiota and function.

The ability of the gut microbiota (the community of bacteria in your gut) to interact with the brain and influence behaviour is becoming a highly interesting notion in the scientific world of health and illness. According to research, your own unique blend of microflora interacts with you as the host to build crucial relationships that regulate the balance and functioning of your entire body. There is no question that the presence of beneficial bacteria in the gut influences brain function. Research has shown that the presence of a specific strain of bacteria known as Bifidobacterium longum NCC3001 eliminates anxiety-like behaviour in mice. Probiotics have been shown to reduce proinflammatory cytokines and increase tryptophan levels, both of which are linked to depression.

The strong link between stress-related psychological symptoms like anxiety and gastrointestinal illnesses like IBD provides additional evidence that the gut-brain axis exists. Poor gut health has been related to a variety of disorders, including ADHD, autism, chronic fatigue, obsessive-compulsive disorder (OCD), Tourette syndrome, and anxiety and depression. Good gut health is unquestionably important for your mental health; once I started paying attention to my gut, my anxiety and melancholy subsided.

Research continues to link gut health to a variety of modern diseases. It appears that Hippocrates was correct all along. The key to intestinal health is found in another of Hippocrates' great statements: "Let food be thy medicine, and medicine be thy food."

You know the truth by the way it feels. Listen to your gut.

FACTORS THAT DAMAGE THE GUT

The prevalence of gut-related health issues during the previous century demonstrates the harmful impact of our post-industrialized diet and lifestyle. Science now reveals that intestinal bacteria mediate a variety of nutritional health consequences, and that diet and lifestyle have a significant impact on the makeup and activity of these bacteria. Leaky gut has been connected to particular nutritional elements in the modern Western lifestyle.

GLUTEN

Gluten-containing grains, notably wheat, are among the most widely consumed foods in the Western world. Wheat and other gluten-containing foods are among the food pyramid's top priorities due to agricultural politics. Whole grains are consistently praised by mainstream media as some of the healthiest foods you can consume for actual health. When it comes to gut health, particularly if it is weakened, consuming wheat or any other gluten-containing meal can cause substantial damage to your intestinal walls.

The Mucosal Biology Research Center at the University of Maryland discovered in 2006 that gliadin (a protein found in wheat's gluten component) can promote intestinal permeability in both celiac and non-celiac mucous membranes. This study demonstrated that wheat gluten triggers signaling via zonulin (a protein involved for altering the shape and permeability of the gut lining) in a way that causes permeable pores in the gut wall. This study found that gliadin leads to intestinal permeability in all individuals, regardless of their autoimmune status caused by gene expression or other causes. In other words, if you want to improve the health of your stomach, you should avoid wheat and all forms of gluten.

The hybridization and recent large use of wheat grain is thought to be one of the primary causes of gluten-induced gastrointestinal issues. The wheat we consume today is very different from the wheat ingested forty years ago. In the 1970s, the ancient bread wheat crop was subjected to extensive hybridization studies in order to address some of the world's hunger issues. The genetically modified wheat grain has significantly higher gluten content and yields ten times more than the traditional Einkorn grain produced in the Middle East.

Unfortunately, this new type of wheat has spread throughout Western agriculture and is now the most common type of wheat available. It provides manufacturers with the highest yield for the lowest price. Unlike the traditional Einkorn grain, it does not grow in nature. It is the outcome of human domestication, intervention, and fertilization. This contemporary wheat has undergone internal and structural changes. Our bodies aren't adapted to this transition, and given wheat's widespread ingestion, this explains the enormous increase in autoimmune disorders in recent decades.

Because wheat is so prevalent in the diets of many people, gluten in all forms should be avoided in order to heal and rebuild your stomach. Gluten is difficult to digest, therefore it deteriorates the gut lining over time, resulting in leaky gut. Gluten leakage in the gut can affect organ function, leading to weariness, fuzzy thinking, anxiety, and sadness, as seen in my personal experience.

FOODS AND OTHER PRODUCTS THAT CONTAIN GLUTEN AND WHEAT

These include:
- baked goods (almost all forms)
- packaged foods and breakfast cereals
- beer
- salami and cured meats
- muesli and muesli bars
- vinegar and soy sauce
- instant meals, frozen foods
- most breads
- baby food
- salad dressings
- sausages
- packaged chips and crackers
- lipstick and cosmetic products

Several chemicals and sweeteners, including glucose syrup, are gluten and wheat-based. If you want to heal and rebuild your gut, avoid all additives. Stick to gluten-free real foods that are free of artificial preservatives and ingredients. I found that eliminating gluten from my diet improved my digestive system and reduced my symptoms significantly. Later on, when your gut has recovered, you can reintroduce gluten into your diet if it suits you.

ANTIBIOTICS

I experienced recurring cystitis before being identified with an autoimmune condition. Each time I had an attack, I would go to the doctor, who would give me a prescription for broad-spectrum antibiotics, which I would diligently take. I feel this led to my autoimmune condition. While antibiotics can be extremely beneficial in treating life-threatening diseases, they are not without risks. Antibiotics are designed to destroy bad bacteria, but they also kill good bacteria. Antibiotic overuse and prescription is thought to have major long-term effects for our health since it has a negative influence on the levels and diversity of our valuable microbiota.

A decrease in healthy bacteria can lead to an excess of harmful bacteria and infections that cause sickness. Antibiotics can cause diarrhoea owing to infections with antibiotic-resistant organisms such salmonella, staphylococcus, and candida, as well as a decrease in beneficial gut flora. If you have an ailment that can be treated without the use of broad-spectrum antibiotics, such as cystitis or the flu (which is caused by a virus that antibiotics can not treat), I recommend that you look into natural recovery options whenever feasible. If antibiotics are essential, a competent integrative doctor or naturopath can provide probiotics and detoxifying herbs like milk thistle to help recolonize your intestines with good bacteria. Steroids (including corticosteroids like prednisone and hydrocortisone), nonsteroidal anti-inflammatory drugs (NSAIDS), antidepressants, laxatives, and antacids are all prescription medications that might alter the equilibrium of your microflora.

INFECTION

Infections with unfriendly microorganisms and bacteria result in an overgrowth of nasty germs, which outnumber the good guys. When hazardous bacteria proliferate in an infection, you may get chronic urinary tract infections, thrush, and yeast infections. When pathogens proliferate and outnumber the beneficial gut flora, it has an impact on overall immunity, which can lead to a cascade of additional issues and infections. The goal is to cultivate a thriving microflora with trillions of cells, promoting a strong immune system, brain, and overall well-being.

STRESS

Stress can be extremely damaging to the health of your stomach. Have you ever had stomach ache before giving a speech? This demonstrates the relationship between the stress reaction and the digestive system. Short-term stress can be manageable, but long-term stress can lead to negative effects such as decreased nutrient absorption, decreased gut oxygenation, four times less blood flow to digestive organs, decreased metabolism, and negative effects on microflora. I have found that including yoga and meditation, as well as establishing a morning routine, are effective approaches to reduce stress. Meditation and deep breathing help to relax the gut and harmonize the gut-brain connection.

EXTERNAL TOXINS

Irritants and toxic compounds that can disrupt gut flora balance and harm the gut lining can take various forms, including processed foods and those containing chemicals, preservatives, flavors, and additives. Avoid artificial sweeteners, nitrites, and cancer-causing foods. Skin, hair, body, and home-care products all contain significant levels of hazardous substances that can cause inside damage.

Chapter 2

Healing and Treatment Protocol

THE FOUR PHASES OF GUT HEALING

Now that you understand how your stomach connects to the rest of your body, it's time to get practical about how you can heal your gut and achieve optimal health. Let's get started with the four steps of gut healing and health improvement.

HEAL YOUR INTESTINAL WALLS

Reduce irritants to your digestive tract. Follow a four-week anti-inflammatory elemental diet to replenish your body with essential nutrients through smoothies, juices, soups, stocks, mashes, and nutritional supplements. Consider your gut as a garden, where you sow seeds, water, and till the soil.

DETOX YOUR BODY

Detoxify your body with oil pulling, Epsom salt baths, dry skin brushing, and gentle movement. Gradually add a natural antibacterial to kill yeasts and bacteria. Cleanse your stomach, detoxify your liver, and gradually reintroduce solid foods. Remove undesirable weeds from your garden to promote healthy plant growth.

START A LONG-TERM HEALTHY DIET

To improve gut health, repopulate it with healthy microflora and consume bacteria-friendly foods. Digestive enzymes can improve digestion and alleviate discomfort. Fertilize your inner garden with probiotic-rich meals.

DETOX YOUR LIFE

To improve your emotional well-being, prioritize self-care, self-love, and gratitude. Plant perennials, annuals, and evergreens to nourish your inner garden and spirit.

Let's break down each process and examine it more closely. The first and most critical step toward a healthy gut is to mend your intestinal walls and establish an environment in which nasty bacteria, candida, and other yeasts cannot thrive or dominate. The plan below will close any permeable pores that may be seeping undigested food into your bloodstream and form a sturdy "net" that will protect your microbiota.

The gut wall serves as a gatekeeper, determining what stays in and what stays out, thus it must be healed and healthy. Fortunately, the small intestine's surface microvilli are extremely regenerative. They can entirely recover in a couple of weeks if they are completely restrained from anything that irritates or inflames them. After restoring my gut health, I saw a significant improvement in my general health. Make changes at your own pace and listen to your body's cues. Don't force something if it doesn't seem right.

This book is simply a guide for you to develop your own healing strategy. Don't be too hard on yourself if you fall off the wagon; it's quite natural to do so and succumb to urges on sometimes. Take each day as it comes, give your body time to heal, and avoid being too hard on yourself.

PHASE ONE: THE ELEMENTAL DIET

GUT-HEALING PROTOCOL

To heal your gut, follow an elemental (liquid) diet for four weeks. This is what I did to heal my gut, and it was absolutely essential to my recovery. A liquid diet refers to healthful, easily digestible meals that the body can absorb, not just juice cleanses or fad diets. This four-week approach entails ingesting liquid meals that still taste good but do not lack nutrition or satiety and are simpler on the digestive system. After extensive research, experimentation, and consultation with integrative doctors and nutritionists, I discovered the most effective way to naturally heal and transform my gut. This allowed my body to heal and strengthen its immune system. After taking a four-week vacation from digesting solid foods, my gut lining mended and became less irritated. This led to improved nutrient absorption, increased energy, and reduced symptoms.

FOODS TO AVOID

The first and most obvious thing I did was to avoid any foods and lifestyle variables that injure the gut and encourage the growth of dangerous bacteria and yeasts. Chapter One's "Factors that damage the gut" goes into greater information about these.

During this time, I also avoided foods that feed nasty bacteria and yeasts, as well as those that caused inflammation in my gut. To determine if a certain meal is causing symptoms, try an elimination diet, even if it's a healthy option. Keep a food diary to track and review your observations. The goal is to give your digestive tract a well-deserved break from difficult-to-digest foods and those that promote inflammation and irritation.

For me, those foods were:

- Any sweetener, sugar, or fruit rich in fructose. This includes honey, agave syrup, maple syrup, refined and unrefined sugar, and all fruits except lemons and limes. Berries are the healthiest option for satisfying your fruit cravings. If they are a problem for you and you see an increase in symptoms, it is best to avoid them for four weeks before reintroducing them once your stomach has healed and your symptoms have subsided.
- Starchy vegetables include beets, carrots, parsnips, potatoes, squash, sweet potatoes, and yams. Cut these out for the first four weeks, then reintroduce them gradually.
- Dairy and milk products in their various forms, including goat and sheep milk. Butter may be used if it does not create symptoms. You can reintroduce goat and sheep milk products after the first four weeks, depending on how you feel.
- Nuts and seeds are fine, however nut milks are acceptable if they do not cause any symptoms. Warm up nut milk to make attractive, soothing, and nourishing drinks.
- All grains, including rice, corn, millet, buckwheat, quinoa, wheat, couscous, amaranth, kamut, spelt, rye, and barley. After healing your stomach, you can reintroduce grains prepared by soaking, sprouting, or fermenting, depending on your personal preferences. Using these preparation methods aids in the breakdown of anti-nutrients (substances that inhibit nutrient absorption), such as phytic acid, making the grains more digestible.
- Beans and lentils are difficult to digest and will just put further strain on your digestive system at this point. They can be consumed later after sprouting and soaking, preferably overnight or for at least eight hours.
- Caffeinated beverages include coffee and chocolate-based drinks. Remove the buzz and relieve the strain on your overworked adrenal glands.

- Caffeine also tricks your tiredness system and reduces healing and detoxifying efforts.
- Bad fats. The most harmful fats and oils to the body include hydrogenated fats (such as trans fats), polyunsaturated fats, and vegetable oils. Hydrogenation produces a highly poisonous substance that is difficult for the body to handle. Avoid vegetable fats and oils such as canola (rapeseed), soy, safflower, sunflower, soybean, and corn oils. Many goods contain fats and oils, including margarine, salad dressings, mayonnaise, and cooking and baking oils. It's also a good idea to learn to read food labels because oils might be combined together.

If you have stomach problems caused by candida overgrowth, you should avoid fermented and fungus-derived foods including soy sauce, tempeh, miso, cheese, mushrooms, alcohol, vinegar, and fermented vegetables. You can reintroduce fermented foods when your gut is ready, but only in small doses and when you can tolerate them.

Once your symptoms have subsided and your gut flora is in balance, you can reintroduce these foods into your diet using the 80/20 rule: eat properly 80% of the time and allow yourself 20% wiggle space.

PHASE TWO: DETOX YOUR BODY

CLEANSE AND SWEEP

As your gut lining heals, you can continue to detox your body. Remember that during the four-week elemental diet, you are still detoxifying your body through the things you eat, especially if you drink enough of water. If you feel up to it, you can begin additional detoxification during week two of the four-week plan, or wait until you are ready. The elemental diet also detoxifies the body, so don't worry if you're not doing everything you can; tiny steps are better than massive ones. Healing, particularly natural healing, takes time and requires patience, especially since your ailment has been present for years. Starting phase two at least two weeks into the four-week elemental diet helps enhance digestion and detoxification.

The rise in symptoms we experience upon starting a detox program is sometimes referred to as a detox reaction or Herxheimer reaction. These reactions occur when the body attempts to expel toxins quicker than they can be appropriately disposed of. Often, you may feel worse, with extra flu-like symptoms and headaches, and believe that the treatment is ineffective. These reactions indicate that the body is purifying itself of impurities, poisons, and imbalances. Increased reactions are transitory and can occur instantly or over a period of days or weeks. In some circumstances, the symptoms are identical to the health conditions you are experiencing, which can be extremely confusing.

The type of detox reaction you'll have will be determined by your overall health or the severity of your current health problem. As old bacteria die and are replaced by new healthy tissue, endotoxins (bacterial toxins) are released into the body. The more severe your body's original state, the more microorganisms exist. Larger amounts of bacteria result in an increased number of endotoxins, and thus a stronger cleansing reaction. This is when it's incredibly vital to relax and attempt to help the detox process along.

STAYING HYDRATED

Maintaining appropriate water and mineral intake is a simple way to minimize or reduce detox effects. Drinking as much water as possible will help to remove toxins from your body. Drinking green juice every day helps your body absorb important nutrients.

Lemon juice with warm water is another hydrating and detoxifying beverage to include in your daily routine. This digestive aid promotes efficient waste elimination, reducing symptoms of indigestion, stomach pain, and bloating. It also helps regulate constipation and diarrhea. Lemon contains powerful antibacterial, antiviral, and immune-boosting properties, as well as the ability to detoxify the liver. Lemons include natural citric acid, calcium, magnesium, copper, folic acid, iron, vitamin B6, vitamin C, and bioflavonoids, which help to boost immunity and fight infection; the juice also works well as a rinse for sore throats and mouth ulcers. They include a high concentration of dietary fiber, which promotes healthy gut bacteria. Consume warm water and lemon on a daily basis to aid in detoxification. To activate your adrenal glands, add a pinch of Celtic sea salt to your morning beverage.

HOW TO MAKE LEMON JUICE IN WARM WATER

Fill the kettle with filtered water, boil it, and then let it cool to a comfortable temperature. Squeeze half a fresh lemon (or 3 tablespoons (60 ml) of freshly squeezed additive-free juice) into a cup or heat-resistant glass, then add water. Wait 20-30 minutes before ingesting. Drink first thing in the morning. Some people like to sip it using a straw because the acid in lemon might damage tooth enamel. If you're out and about, most restaurants and cafés will accommodate you if you want hot water and lemonade.

DRY SKIN BRUSHING

Spend a few minutes scrubbing your dry skin before taking a morning shower or bath. This Ayurvedic lifestyle staple aids in the detoxification and elimination of pollutants via the skin, the body's largest and most important eliminative organ. The skin is normally the last organ in the body to receive nutrients, but it is the first to show signs of an imbalance or deficit. Dry skin brushing stimulates the lymphatic system by facilitating the movement of lymph throughout the body. It stimulates the liver and adrenal glands, allowing them to decongest and eliminate toxins.

Dry skin brushing provides numerous benefits. It:

- Improves digestion and renal function, and promotes cell repair and rejuvenation.
- Encourages the body to release metabolic wastes.
- Stimulates acupressure points.
- Helps your skin absorb nutrients.
- Boosts the immune system
- Improves muscular tone and even distribution of fat deposits.
- Removes dead skin cells and external contaminants.
- Stimulates and enhances blood circulation.
- Aids the elimination capability of your body's organs.

STEP-BY-STEP GUIDE TO DRY SKIN BRUSHING

Purchase a long-handled bath brush with natural bristles (avoid synthetic bristles, which can harm the skin and be harsh and unpleasant). The brush should be kept dry and used once on each part of your body excluding your face. There is no need to scrub; instead, use lengthy strokes that go back and forth in a circle. Brush only toward the heart. To keep the brush fresh, wash it with soap and water every few weeks and let it to dry naturally. Loofahs can also be used.

- Brush first thing in the morning, before taking a shower. Ensure that your skin and brush are fully dry.
- Begin with the soles of your feet, then move up both sides of your legs. Next, brush your back, then move on to your abdomen, working clockwise in the direction of your colon. Then, proceed up toward your heart, being cautious of the chest region.
- Avoid brushing your face because it is a sensitive area.
- Start with mild strokes to become acquainted to the sensation. Your skin should feel stimulated and tingly, but not inflamed or red.

- Take a shower to eliminate dirt and dead skin cells.

HOW TO REST INTENTIONALLY

Find a quiet place to make your meditation session memorable. Sit or lie down in a comfortable position and focus on the part of your body that is causing you anxiety, discomfort, pain, or inflammation. When you focus your awareness and attention on a specific part of your body or mind, your body will automatically tense up. That's how we're used to dealing with pain. To relieve pain, take deep breaths into your belly and imagine yourself resting the affected area of your body. Don't try to fix it; instead, intentionally let it rest.

Do this exercise wherever and whenever you are in pain. It will allow you to truly rest and regenerate energy in that area. Bingo!

SET YOUR INTENTION

Before we begin, let's get in the appropriate mindset and make an intention to actually promote healing. Remember, stress is one of the reasons that contribute to an unhappy gut, so attempt to reduce any stressors in your life. It's also time to trust your instincts and start flexing your "Mr or Mrs No" muscles. That could entail declining individuals or invitations and putting your people pleasing inclinations on hold, both personally and professionally.

It's time to prioritize self-care and nourishment in order to preserve your most valuable resource: yourself! To begin, set your desire to heal, and then trust your instincts.

Sometimes the most productive thing to do is to give yourself a break and enjoy the pleasure of missing out. I understand how difficult it is when you have a family, a job, and obligations, yet being a rebel can be rewarding. Begin by establishing some new ground rules that will help you conserve your energy. This allows you to refuel and renew. Make an attempt to turn off your computer, electronics, and screens and take some time off. Rest is vital for your overall health and might help you repair your gut faster.

OIL PULLING

Oil pulling is a vital therapeutic activity to incorporate during the first four weeks and beyond. Oil pulling is a traditional Ayurvedic practice that has been linked to improved health, including digestive issues. The procedure has a tremendous detoxifying impact, eradicating yeasts, harmful bacteria, parasites, fungus, and viruses in the mouth, including candida and streptococci. Killing bacteria in the mouth prevents subsequent infections in the gut, which can lead to many disorders throughout the body.

Kavala and gandusa are the two oil-pulling techniques used in Ayurvedic medicine. When practicing kavala, you fill your mouth with liquid, close it, and hold the liquid in for a few minutes. After that, you begin swirling the liquid about your mouth before spitting it out.

The procedure should not take more than three or four minutes and is performed two or three times. Gandusa is a separate technique that involves holding the liquid in the mouth for three to five minutes without swishing it around. You then spit out the liquid and repeat the procedure.

To oil pull with coconut oil, simply place 1 tablespoon (20 ml) of extra virgin cold-pressed coconut oil in your mouth upon rising. It is best done on an empty stomach and before consuming any liquids. Swish the oil around your mouth for 10-20 minutes before spitting it.

Never consume the oil, which contains microorganisms. Brush your teeth well afterward to eliminate any remaining oil. To avoid nasty bacteria buildup, acquire a toothbrush designed specifically for oil pulling and carefully clean it with a 3 percent hydrogen peroxide solution.

Including this easy habit in your daily routine will bring additional benefits such as whiter teeth, cleaner skin, healthier gums, fresher breath, clearer sinuses, better regulated menstrual cycles, an improved lymphatic system, better sleep, and more vitality. This simple yet effective activity offers numerous health benefits. It is well worth the swoosh!

SUPERCHARGED TIP

Epsom salts absorb excess oil from hair and can be added to your preferred shampoo when it is overly oily. Add around 1/4 cup (2 fl oz/60 ml) when shampooing. To condition your hair naturally, use lemon juice as a rinse.

EPSOM SALTS BATHS

Make time for yourself to take an Epsom salt bath at least twice a week. Bathing with Epsom salts absorbs magnesium sulfate via the skin, effectively removing toxins. It relaxes the nervous system, lowers swelling, loosens muscles, soothes pain, and acts as a natural emollient and exfoliant.

HOW TO MAKE AN EPSOM SALTS BATH

The ideal approach to make an Epsom salts bath is to pour 2 cups (17 oz/500 ml) into a warm bath while it is running. Once the bath is at the appropriate level and temperature for you, slowly jump in and soak for 15-20 minutes.

MORE GREAT DETOX TECHNIQUES

If you have access to one, try visiting a sauna or steam room to relax your muscles while also encouraging sweating and detoxification through the skin. This treatment method enhances circulation and cleanses the body. Heat has an analgesic, or pain-relieving impact on the body. It also helps you relax and unwind while reducing muscle tension.

Saltwater flushes and enemas can also help the body detoxify.

PHASE THREE: MAINTAIN AND RESTORE WITH FOOD

After you've finished the four-week elemental diet and restored and rebalanced your gut bacteria with natural antibiotics and antimicrobials, your gut will have had a much-needed break, repairing and recovering from permeable holes and inflammation in your digestive tract. Your gut lining can now provide a safe "home" for your gut bacteria to survive, thrive, and fight off any bad guys that may enter your stomach.

To enhance your immune system, control hormones, and increase cognitive function, feed healthy gut flora after repairing the gut lining and eradicating harmful bacteria. There are numerous foods and substances you may now incorporate to help establish this healthy community. Consider your gut to be a garden that can only bloom in healthy soil. Healthy soil necessitates healthy meals and nutrients, which will enable the "good guys" to thrive.

But first, you must make a small, lifetime commitment to gut health and upkeep. Health cannot be obtained by a quick-fix diet or a simple prescription; it requires you to make good decisions every day. After completing the four-week gut-healing treatment, cleanse, and sweep, you can continue to enhance your gut health over the next four weeks (or as needed).

EVERYDAY CHECKLIST

CUT DOWN OR ELIMINATE GLUTEN

- Based on what we know about gluten's influence on intestinal permeability, it's reasonable to say you should avoid it if you want to continue restoring gut health. Instead of eating gluten-filled grains, choose for unprocessed gluten-free

- grains like buckwheat, quinoa, and brown rice.

GO EASY ON SUGAR
- Too much evidence shows how bad sugar is for our health. Bad bacteria love an excess of sugar to feast on, which includes overindulging in fruit. Avoid any refined white sugar, which is the worst sort. To replace sugar, consider adding stevia, rice malt syrup, or fruit to enhance sweetness. When consuming fruit, limit yourself to one piece per day, or select for low-fructose options like berries, lemons, limes, and grapefruit.

GET CRAZY WITH VEGETABLES
- Your gut craves easy-to-digest foods, and plant foods are soft on the stomach. Consume plenty of chlorophyll-rich greens, vegetable juices, and earthy vegetarian soups made from prebiotic-rich root vegetables to keep your good bacteria nourished with antioxidants, enzymes, and nutrients for proper digestion.

CONSUME FERMENTED FOODS DAILY
- Once your gut lining has healed, and you are ready, you can begin to incorporate one cultured food, such as Cultured Vegetables, Easy-to-Make Sauerkraut, Kimchi, Coconut Kefir, or Homemade Kombucha, to colonize your gut with healthy flora and boost your inner ecosystem. When first starting off with fermented foods, consume only a fourth of the suggested amount per serving, or begin with just one teaspoon and work your way up. Eating a range of various fermented foods will contribute a variety of bacterial strains, which will supply the diversity needed for a healthy microbiome.

DRINK PLENTY OF PURE, FILTERED WATER
- Water is essential for gut health because it helps wash out pollutants; however, normal tap water contains fluoride and chlorine, both of which are harmful to microflora. Choose to invest in an excellent water filter and consume at least eight glasses every day. Adding lemon juice or apple cider vinegar to water improves digestion, breaks up mucus, frees up the lymphatic system, and boosts immunity.

WHEN IN DOUBT REMEMBER WHOLE FOODS
- Based on everything I've said, it's clear that the best way to achieve optimal health is to eat foods in their most natural form. The more nature is disrupted in your diet, the less likely your gut bacteria will be able

- to tolerate it. Eat foods that are natural and unprocessed. Wherever feasible, opt for organic and chemical-free products. Consume grass-fed meat and animal products in the quantities that would be naturally available if mass meat production did not exist. Incorporate more plant-based foods into your diet. Eating this way will offer you with all the nutrients your digestive system requires to function optimally, giving healing nutrients to all of your body's systems.

REINTRODUCING FOOD

By now, you'll be delighted to see your symptoms fade and feel better with more energy, cleaner skin, and better digestion. However, for some of you, the prospect of resuming food may be daunting.

You had a nutritional blueprint to follow for the first few phases of the procedure, so you knew what to eat and when, how to get organized, and what to do while detoxing. But now it's time to reintroduce food; you may be wondering what you should eat or whether your symptoms may return once you resume regular eating. I hear you.

The change can be difficult, and it's tempting to revert to bad habits as soon as you feel better. Of course, staying on a liquid diet indefinitely is inconvenient, but you also cannot immediately return to your old eating habits. To maintain the benefits of the program and live a healthy, fulfilling life with a restored gut, it's important to gradually and carefully reintroduce foods.

The next several weeks are essential because your gut is still susceptible, and when you resume normal eating, you must proceed gently and pay close attention to what your body tells you. But first, let's define "normal eating". I'm not sure about your previous eating habits, but I didn't comprehend the impact of food on my health until I became ill. After completing the elemental diet, I became so conscious of the effects of food on my body, both positive and negative, that I changed my perspective on food and nutrition permanently. Limiting gluten, sugar, and dairy is effective for me, but individual needs may vary.

I'm not suggesting you to eat exactly as I do, but I do encourage you to be interested and open to trying new foods, experimenting with different recipes and habits, and observing how your body feels. Consuming healthy, gut-friendly cuisine as a new way of eating does not have to be monotonous, expensive, or time-consuming. You don't need advanced cooking abilities, expensive equipment, or a personal chef. Once you've experimented with a few recipes and become acquainted with the ingredients, you'll discover that healthy eating can be both enjoyable and tasty! Eating natural whole foods is essential for a healthy gut and body, but it doesn't mean you can't indulge occasionally.

In my life, I apply the 80/20 rule. I eat healthy, gut-friendly foods 80 percent of the time and indulge in my favorite pleasures 20% of the time. Remember that you are defined by what you do on a consistent basis, not what you do occasionally. Nowadays, my treats are largely healthy, such as handmade chocolate and muffins, but I still enjoy gelato!

If you're wanting your grandmother's carrot cake or can't resist a slice of pizza at a dinner party, it's okay to indulge! But don't forget to enjoy it. Enjoy every bite with mindfulness. And most importantly: Don't feel guilty. Guilt causes stress reactions in your body that are far worse for your gut than the gluten in pizza or the sugar in carrot cake! It's perfectly fine to indulge in and enjoy goodies.

And after a while, when sustaining your body with nutritious foods becomes a habit, you'll feel so good that you won't crave that slice of cake or pizza.

However, before you may enjoy your favorite delicacies on sometimes, you must gradually reintroduce food and pay great attention to your body's response.

This could be the ideal time to try an elimination diet. This basically means that you exclude particular meals for a set length of time, usually three or four weeks, and then gradually reintroduce them one by one while monitoring your symptoms. There are many different versions of the elimination diet, but they all recommend avoiding gluten, dairy, soy, eggs, and maize. Other typical irritating foods to avoid include pork, beans and lentils, caffeine, nuts and seeds, and nightshade vegetables.

At the end of the elimination period, choose one of the foods you avoided, such as gluten or dairy, and eat it (but not in excess). Consider how you feel during the next 48 hours. If you have no reaction after two days, consume the same food again and watch for any reactions. Based on how you feel, you can determine whether to reinstate that food into your diet on a regular basis.

Next, choose another dish and repeat the process. Throughout the diet and reintroduction phase, you must pay great attention to how you feel and record any physical, mental, or emotional symptoms. Keep a meal log and track your sleep, mood, energy, digestion, and skin. Take note, for example, if you suffer from sleeplessness, exhaustion, joint discomfort, skin breakouts or rashes, headaches, changes in bowel movements, bloating, brain fog, or sinus problems.

The entire procedure will take five to eight weeks, depending on how many items you've removed, but by the end of the experiment, you'll have learned a lot about how your body reacts to different foods. It's a tremendously empowering tool to be your own health investigator and determine what's best for your body. To reintroduce solid foods after the elemental diet, begin with steamed vegetables and soft meals like casseroles, slow-cooked entrees, and steamed fish or poultry served with brown rice, buckwheat, or quinoa. If an elimination diet is not desired, this is the best option.

Include easy-to-digest foods so that your gut can gradually adjust to digesting solid food. I advocate setting aside two days per week to solely eat liquids or to fast intermittently. This is especially useful during the first few weeks while you're adjusting to eating solid meals again. Reintroduce raw foods slowly. They demand more effort from your digestive system to process, so give your body plenty of time to adjust to digesting them again.

As you can see, I'm not providing you a rigid diet or a ten page list of foods to avoid because we're all unique. You may thrive on dairy products, whilst someone else may get severe symptoms from just one glass of milk! I encourage you to be your own leader and discover what works for your body. It is a trial-and-error procedure, so be patient. But it's also incredibly satisfying and empowering.

SUPERCHARGED TIP

Life isn't about being perfect or dogmatic. This will increase stress and be detrimental to the situation. Listen to your body, be gentle, and do what feels best for you.

PREBIOTICS

Some argue that the statement "You are what you eat" should be "You are what your bacteria eat." Did you know that your beneficial bacteria require specific foods to survive? As previously stated, these foods are classed as prebiotics. They are the precise nutrients that nourish your beneficial microorganisms. More specifically, they are meals containing non-digestible but fermentable oligosaccharides that alter the structure and activity of your gut flora, with the goal of improving the health of their host (you!).

Instead of using problematic prebiotic

supplements, it's critical to consume a variety of fiber-rich foods to complement your diet with prebiotics. Garlic, for example, is an excellent prebiotic meal because it not only kills harmful bacteria but also contains dietary fructins, which are prebiotics that feed specific strains of bacteria that are beneficial to your health.

Foods high in soluble fiber are broken down in the large intestine into a gelatinous, viscous byproduct that creates acids and gasses that encourage the growth of beneficial microorganisms. Soluble fiber-rich foods such as sweet potatoes, brussels sprouts, asparagus, turnips, mangoes, avocados, strawberries, and apricots are excellent prebiotics.

Resistant starches are those that remain undigested until they reach the large intestine, where they are digested similarly to soluble and insoluble fibers. Potatoes, lentils, nuts, and seeds all contain resistant starch. Remember to slowly reintroduce these foods into your diet and observe how your stomach reacts.

PHASE FOUR
DETOX YOUR LIFE

Now that you've cleansed your stomach, it's time to detox your emotions, your home, and the products you use on your skin. Food alone will not guarantee a strong colony of beneficial bacteria in your stomach. Even the best diet can be undone by stress and emotions.

Stress can be acute or chronic. Chronic, long-term stress that lasts for weeks is extremely bad for gut health. Stress generates a variety of reactions in the gut, including changes in gastric secretions, gut motility, mucosal permeability, visceral (or organ) sensitivity, and barrier function. Evidence also reveals that negative emotions and stress have a harmful impact on our gut microbes. Stress hormones promote the growth of harmful microorganisms.

What is it that makes you stressed? The objective is to identify the underlying reason. Is it something you can control? What lifestyle adjustments or actions can you make to reduce stress in your life? If the answer is uncertain, exercises like yoga, walking, and swimming can help alleviate these symptoms. When was the last time you went outside into the sunshine and interacted with nature? Sunlight and bare feet on the ground (known as earthing) have a therapeutic effect on hormones and the brain. A combination of these lifestyle modifications, including a wholefoods diet, may be enough to alleviate your symptoms.

Toxic relationships and friendships may be keeping you from obtaining inner peace and gut health. Choose to surround oneself with good and nice people. You'll feel greater delight by purifying your relationships and engaging in mutually life-giving interpersonal connections, which your gut bacteria will appreciate.

Meditation is another excellent activity that can help you control your thoughts and emotions. While it involves discipline, it has been demonstrated to have significant benefits for emotional health and stress. Develop a grateful mindset by identifying three things to be thankful for every morning and reflecting on them.

Did you know that giving back to your community is another strategy to reduce stress and improve your mental health? Giving to others can enhance our emotional well-being. It also improves social connections and has been proved to increase life expectancy!

What is it that causes you stress? Figuring out the cause is the key. Is it something you can control? What lifestyle changes or decisions can you make to remove stress from your life?

If stress and negative thought patterns are a larger issue for you, counseling and psychology may be required, and that is fine! Addressing any remaining emotional difficulties is critical for your health. The relationship between your stomach and your emotions is reciprocal. They both have the potential to have a negative impact on one another, therefore it is critical to manage your mental health as well as the food you consume.

YOUR HEALTHY HOME

Maintaining a healthy gut requires minimizing your toxic load. Toxins and chemicals inhaled or absorbed through the skin must be dealt with by your gut immune system. Taking the pressure off the good guys will allow them to complete all of the health-promoting tasks on their to-do list. This entails removing poisons and hazardous compounds wherever possible.

Chemicals in household cleaning products have been related to a variety of ailments. Triclosan, a common chemical in antibacterial hand soap, has been related to hormonal disturbance and is a recognized carcinogen. Replace harmful products with simple, handmade, or chemical-free alternatives, and discard those with unfamiliar constituents.

Almost all chemical-based cleaning

products can be substituted with three ingredients: baking soda, white vinegar, and lemon juice. They will eliminate hazardous microorganisms and leave your home spotless with no negative side effects.

You're now making the transition to a healthier lifestyle. Check for yoga. Check for daily green juice. Buying organic produce: check, check, check. Have you considered the dangerous pollutants present in your furniture, upholstery, and mattress?

These dangerous pollutants are referred to as volatile organic compounds (VOCs). VOCs are carbon-based compounds that evaporate or easily enter the atmosphere at ambient temperature. This is the odor you could notice after the carpets have been thoroughly cleaned or when the walls have been freshly painted. Not all VOCs have a strong odor; some have none at all but inflict the same amount of harm to the body. Potential side effects include headaches, dizziness, nausea, and eye/nose/throat irritation. Long-term exposure to these chemicals can cause them to accumulate in your body, raising the risk of liver and kidney damage.

Common VOCs include formaldehyde, benzene, acetone, and ethylene glycol, which can be found in air fresheners, paint, varnish, upholstery fabrics, vinyl, cosmetics, and moth balls. Common floor coverings, as well as all forms of synthetic carpets, carpet underlay, and upholstery made of synthetic foams, foam rubber, latex, or plastic, are frequently the principal sources of indoor air contamination. This is because they either contain VOCs or are present in the adhesives used to install them.

Furniture and carpets with chemical finishes, such as stain repellents and brominated flame retardants, are also hazardous. Avoid recarpeting or pulling out your carpets while pregnant.

Bedroom furnishings also contain chemicals, such as flame retardants and stain repellents. These can be found in most foam mattresses, synthetic drapes, upholstery, and carpets. Even dry-cleaned garments produce harmful substances!

Avoid storing too many electrical and electronic appliances in your bedroom at the same time, such as computers, televisions, and hi-fi systems, as these are also treated with brominated flame retardants.

Mold is a major indoor air polluter that can occur at any time of year in wet regions of a home or apartment, particularly in south-facing rooms. Poorly managed air-conditioning systems can potentially spread mold throughout the home.

HOW TO CREATE A HEALTHY HOME

- Choose your furnishings intelligently; natural finishes such as oils, waxes, and polishes are preferable to polyurethane, varnishes, melamine, or paint, all of which generate VOCs.
- When repainting, select low-VOC or natural paints. Paint can be a substantial source of interior air pollution, especially when it is newly applied. If your paint is over 45 years old, it may contain significant levels of lead. Check for flaking and lead dust.
- Make sure your gas heaters are flued (and cleaned). An unflued gas heater can produce hazardous fumes.
- Reduce the impact of cleaning goods by using low-harm alternatives such as vinegar instead of bleach. Cleaning the house on a regular basis is essential for maintaining a healthy home.
- To remove dirt and mold, open your windows and doors on a regular basis.
- Instead of using artificial air fresheners, open your windows as wide as possible. If you can't keep the windows open, apply natural odor removers. A bowl of baking soda can easily absorb odors. Alternatively, utilize natural fragrances like potpourri or lavender, or better yet, burn essential oils to boost the positive effects.
- Vacuum with a HEPA filter machine to keep dust mites away.
- Indoor plants can act as natural air filters, cleaning the air of VOCs and other contaminants.
- Keep a doormat at the front or back door to prevent dirt and pollutants from being tracked throughout the house, or require residents to remove their shoes before leaving the dirt at the door.
- Choose carpets made of natural fibers like wool, cotton, rattan, or jute. Not only do they look and feel better, but they are also safer for you and the environment.
- Choose drapes, carpets, and upholstery that contain minimal or no brominated flame retardants or stain repellents.
- When purchasing a PC or monitor, search for the TCO'95 Ecolabel, which specifies the amount of brominated flame retardant in the product.
- If you've recently redecorated your home or moved into a newly decorated one, airing it out will neutralize the chemicals when they're at their most effective. However, high levels of VOCs will continue to

- emit for months, if not years.
- It's difficult to live in a bubble and avoid every dangerous chemical you come into touch with, so phase them out at your own pace and as needed to fit into your lifestyle.

DETOX YOUR SKIN

The skin is a digestive organ, with 60% of anything you put on it being absorbed directly into your circulation. When you think about it, nicotine patches are designed to be applied on the skin so that nicotine can be absorbed into the body; why wouldn't the components you apply to your skin on a daily basis leach into your system as well? This is scary, given that the average woman uses around 515 chemicals on her skin each day.

The beauty industry loves to market the promise of endless youth, skyscraper lashes, and a sun-kissed glow, yet many frightening truths lurk beneath these promises of beauty and charm. More than 10,000 chemical compounds are now approved for use in personal care products. Pick one of those moisturizers off the shelf the next time you go shopping and read the ingredients label; you'll no longer be amazed that this is the case. Chemicals have been connected to various diseases and body reactions, posing a risk.

Common skincare components such as sodium lauryl sulfate, polyethylene glycol, parabens, isopropyl myristate, and phthalates have been associated to a wide range of diseases, including immune system disorders, allergies, cancer, and infertility. Toxins can be exhausting for your intestines.

Taking these facts into consideration, it is critical that you read the ingredient lists of your products and conduct research to ensure that you and your family are protected from their harmful effects. Organic bath, beauty, and skincare products should be free of synthetic preservatives, toxins, artificial perfumes, colors, and mineral oils. I personally removed every contaminant from my beauty routine, including my daily lotions and potions.

Once you've refilled your makeup bag and bathroom cupboards with safe, organic items, you'll notice an increase in your general health, which will improve your appearance in the long run.
Never be duped by the cosmetics industry's extravagant boasts.

There is no doubt that beauty stems mostly from within. It is a major mistake to believe that piling ingredients on the outside of our bodies will make us beautiful. By nourishing your body with colorful, antioxidant-rich, chemical-free meals and healthy fats, you could foster a healthy, thriving colony of bacteria, resulting in a natural, glowing appearance.

Chapter 3

Appetizers and Snacks

Brazilian Cheesy Bread

- **MAKES 24 2-INCH ROLLS**

Ingredients
- 1 cup goat's milk, casein A2 milk, or unsweetened coconut milk
- ½ cup avocado oil
- 1 teaspoon iodized sea salt
- 10 ounces (about 2 cups) cassava flour
- 2 large omega-3 or pastured eggs or Vegan Eggs
- 1 to 1½ cups grated Parmigiano-Reggiano cheese, or 1 cup nutritional yeast

Directions
- Preheat your oven to 450°F and place two evenly spaced racks inside.
- Prepare two baking sheets using parchment paper or silicone baking mats.
- Pour the milk, oil, and salt into a medium pot. Bring to a simmer on medium heat, stirring occasionally.
- Remove from heat when large bubbles appear.
- Add the cassava flour to the saucepan and whisk with a wooden spoon until thoroughly blended. A gelatinous dough will start to develop.
- Transfer the dough to the bowl of a stand mixer equipped with the paddle attachment. Beat the dough on medium speed for a few minutes until it appears smooth and cool enough to touch comfortably.
- Beat the eggs into the cooled mixture one at a time with the mixer set to medium speed. Wait until the first egg is completely integrated before adding the second. Scrape the edges of the bowl frequently to achieve even mixing.
- If using cheese, beat it in at medium speed. You'll have a flexible, sticky dough that's softer than cookie dough but firmer than cake batter.
- Scoop the dough with a small ice cream scoop and equally distribute it on the baking sheets (approximately 12 per sheet). Dip the scoop in a dish

- of water between scoops to prevent dough from sticking.
- Place the baking sheets in the oven and lower the temperature to 350°F. Bake for 15 minutes, then switch the baking sheets.
- Bake for a further 10-15 minutes, or until the bread is brown. Remove from the oven and let cool for a few minutes before serving.

Nutritional Information Per Roll (1 of 24):
- Calories: ~110
- Protein: ~2-3 g
- Fat: ~7 g
- Carbohydrates: ~10 g
- Sodium: ~150-200 mg

Avocado Deviled Eggs

MAKES 12

Ingredients
- 6 omega-3 or pastured eggs, hard-boiled and peeled
- 1 ripe avocado, skin and seed removed
- 1 tablespoon Dijon mustard
- 1 teaspoon grated horseradish
- 1 teaspoon iodized sea salt
- Juice of 1 lemon
- Paprika, to garnish

Directions

- Cut the eggs in half lengthwise and scoop out the yolks, placing them in the work bowl of a food processor.
- In the food processor bowl, combine the avocado, mustard, horseradish, sea salt, and lemon juice. Blend until smooth.
- Return the yolk mixture to the egg whites and finish with a sprinkle of paprika.

Nutritional Information Per Serving (1 of 12):
- Calories: ~60
- Protein: ~3 g
- Fat: ~5 g
- Saturated Fat: ~1 g
- Carbohydrates: ~1 g
- Sodium: ~90 mg

Dr. Gundry's Nut Mix 2.0

SERVES 12 TO 15

Ingredients
- 1 cup raw walnuts
- 1 cup raw pistachios
- ½ cup raw pecans
- ½ cup raw macadamia nuts
- 2 tablespoons extra-virgin olive oil
- 2 cloves garlic, minced
- 2 tablespoons fresh rosemary, minced
- 1 teaspoon paprika
- 1 teaspoon iodized sea salt

Directions
- Place nuts in a large basin and set aside.
- In a small sauté pan, heat olive oil over medium heat. Add the garlic and rosemary and simmer for 2 to 3 minutes, or until fragrant.
- Remove from heat and quickly pour oil mixture over nut mix, followed by paprika and sea salt.
- Toss to blend, then serve.

Nutritional Information: Per Serving (based on 15 servings):
- Calories: ~190
- Protein: ~4 g
- Fat: ~18 g
- Saturated Fat: ~2 g
- Carbohydrates: ~4 g
- Fiber: ~2 g
- Sodium: ~160 mg

Broccoli Puffs

MAKES ABOUT 20

Ingredients
- 2 cups broccoli florets, steamed until tender
- 1 egg or VeganEgg
- ½ yellow onion, minced
- 1 clove garlic, minced
- ½ cup cassava flour
- ¼ cup blanched almond meal
- ½ teaspoon black pepper
- ½ teaspoon yacón syrup or local honey
- 1 teaspoon iodized sea salt
- 1 tablespoon minced parsley
- ¼ cup grated Parmigiano-Reggiano cheese or nutritional yeast
- Hot sauce for dipping (optional)

Directions
- Preheat the oven to 400° Fahrenheit. Grease a baking sheet with a thin layer of oil and put aside.
- In a food processor fitted with an S-blade, combine the broccoli, egg, onion, garlic, cassava flour, almond meal, pepper, syrup or honey, salt, parsley, and cheese or yeast.
- Scoop roughly one and a half tablespoons of the mixture and press lightly between your palms to make a tater-tot shape. To avoid sticking, wash your hands every few tots. Place the tots on a baking sheet, evenly spaced.
- Bake for 18–20 minutes, or until golden brown. Serve with hot sauce or guacamole, if desired.

Nutritional Information: Per Puff (1 of 20):
- Calories: ~35
- Protein: ~1 g
- Fat: ~1.5 g
- Carbohydrates: ~4 g
- Fiber: ~1 g
- Sodium: ~90 mg

Caramelized Onion Dip

SERVES 6 TO 8

Ingredients
- 2 tablespoons extra-virgin olive oil
- 2 large yellow onions, thinly sliced
- 1 clove garlic, minced
- 1 tablespoon fresh thyme leaves
- 1 teaspoon fresh rosemary, minced
- 1 teaspoon iodized sea salt
- 1 teaspoon ground black pepper
- Zest of 1 lemon
- Juice of 1 lemon
- 2 cups plain coconut yogurt
- Minced chives, to garnish
- 1 jicama, peeled and cut into sticks

Directions
- In a large pan, warm the olive oil over medium-low heat. Add the onions and cook for 8 minutes, stirring frequently, until tender and translucent.
- Add the garlic, thyme, rosemary, sea salt, pepper, and lemon zest, and simmer for 10 to 15 minutes, stirring occasionally, until the onions are evenly browned. (If the garlic begins to brown, reduce the heat to low.)
- Stir in the lemon juice, then remove the pan from the heat and allow to cool completely.
- Stir the coconut yogurt into the cooled onion mixture until well mixed. Transfer the dip to a serving dish and sprinkle with chives. Serve alongside jicama sticks, other fresh vegetables, chips, or crackers.

Nutritional Information: Per Serving (based on 8 servings):
- Calories: ~80
- Protein: ~1 g
- Fat: ~5 g
- Saturated Fat: ~3 g
- Carbohydrates: ~7 g
- Fiber: ~1 g
- Sodium: ~250 mg

Cassava Tortillas (and Chips)

MAKES 10 LARGE OR 18 SMALL TORTILLAS

Ingredients
- 2 cups cassava flour
- 1 cup unsweetened coconut milk or goat's milk
- ½ cup avocado oil
- ½ cup water
- 2 teaspoons iodized sea salt
- Olive oil, ghee, or avocado oil, for cooking

Directions

TO MAKE TORTILLAS
- In a medium mixing bowl, combine the cassava flour, milk, avocado oil,

- salt, and water. Mix with a wooden spoon until well mixed. The dough should have a smooth and cohesive texture.
- Divide the dough into 10 bigger or 18 smaller equal portions and form into balls. On a sheet of parchment paper, roll each part into a slightly thicker-than-average tortilla. (If you own a tortilla press, feel free to use it instead.) If the dough sticks to the rolling pin, add a little coating of cassava flour.
- Preheat a frying pan on the stove over medium-low heat. Brush the skillet with oil or ghee, then cook the tortillas for 3 to 4 minutes per side.
- Serve immediately, unless converting into chips.

TO MAKE CHIPS

- Preheat the oven to 425° Fahrenheit. Brush oil onto a sheet tray and leave aside.
- Brush avocado oil on both sides of tortillas and cut into chip-sized wedges.
- Place in a single layer on the baking sheet and bake for 10 to 15 minutes, until crispy.
- Serve alongside Plant Paradox Guacamole.

NOTE: These are not as easy to handle as flour tortillas; they are quite fragile. So, be careful when moving them to the pan and flipping them, as they tend to fracture.

I find it easier to make little tortillas until you get used to working with this delicate dough.

Chips Three Ways

Sweet Potato Chips

Ingredients
- 1 Japanese sweet potato, peeled
- 2 to 3 cups avocado oil or extra-virgin olive oil
- 2 tablespoons iodized sea salt

Directions
- Use a vegetable peeler to slice the sweet potato into thin slices.
- Cover the bottom of a big skillet with 1 to 2 inches of oil.
- Heat the oil on medium until "shimmering."
- Saute the sweet potato slices till golden brown on one side. Flip and repeat.
- Place the golden chips on a paper towel and season with salt.
- Repeat until all the slices are golden brown.

Plantain Chips

Ingredients
- 2 green plantains, peeled and thinly sliced
- 1½ tablespoons olive oil
- ¾ teaspoon salt
- Freshly ground pepper to taste

Directions
- Preheat the oven to 400° Fahrenheit. Put parchment paper on a cookie sheet and put aside.
- Toss plantain pieces, olive oil, and seasonings in a bowl.
- Spread the plantains in a single layer on the prepared cookie sheet.
- Bake for 15 to 20 minutes, flipping plantains halfway through (about 8 minutes).
- When the plantain chips begin to brown around the edges, remove from the oven immediately.

Prosciutto Chips

Ingredients
- 10 thin slices pasture-raised prosciutto

Directions
- Preheat the oven to 350° Fahrenheit. Put parchment paper on a cookie sheet.
- Place the prosciutto slices in a single layer on a cookie sheet fitted with paper.
- Bake until crispy, about 5 to 7 minutes. Allow them to cool (they become crisper when chilled).
- Break them into tiny pieces and serve as a topper for any entrée, salad, or on their own. They are quite addictive!

Buffalo Cauliflower Bites

SERVES 4 TO 6

Ingredients

FOR THE BUFFALO SAUCE
- ½ cup Frank's Red Hot Sauce
- 2½ teaspoons avocado oil or ghee
- 1 tablespoon coconut aminos
- 1 teaspoon apple cider vinegar
- 1 medium head of cauliflower, chopped
- 2 tablespoons extra-virgin olive oil, plus more for baking sheet
- 2 tablespoons cassava flour
- 1 teaspoon iodized sea salt
- 1 teaspoon ground black pepper
- 2 teaspoons garlic powder
- ½ cup buffalo sauce
- Plain coconut yogurt, for dipping

Directions
- Preheat the oven to 450° Fahrenheit.
- To prepare the buffalo sauce, put the hot sauce, avocado oil or ghee, coconut aminos, and apple cider vinegar in a glass container with a cover and shake vigorously. Refrigerate until needed.
- Drizzle olive oil liberally on a baking sheet or line it with paper. Set aside.
- In a large mixing bowl, combine the cauliflower, olive oil, cassava flour, and spices and toss to coat evenly

- Transfer to a baking sheet and bake for 30 minutes, rotating every 10 minutes until the cauliflower is crisp on all sides.
- Brush with buffalo sauce and bake for an additional 10 minutes.
- Serve with yogurt and any remaining buffalo sauce for dipping.

Nutritional Information: Per Serving (based on 6 servings):
- Calories: ~100
- Protein: ~2 g
- Fat: ~7 g
- Saturated Fat: ~1 g
- Carbohydrates: ~9 g
- Fiber: ~2 g
- Sodium: ~500 mg

Garlic-and-Walnut-Stuffed Mushrooms

SERVES 12

Ingredients
- 12 bite-size brown mushrooms, such as cremini, wiped with a damp towel
- ¼ cup plus 2 tablespoons extra-virgin olive oil
- ½ brown onion, minced
- 4 cloves garlic
- 1 teaspoon fresh thyme
- 1 cup diced walnuts
- ½ teaspoon salt
- ½ teaspoon poultry seasoning
- ½ teaspoon paprika
- ¼ cup coconut cream
- ¼ cup minced parsley, to garnish (optional)

Directions
- Remove the stems from the mushrooms to prepare them. Crumble the stems and set aside.
- In a large, lidded skillet, heat 2 tablespoons olive oil. When the oil is shimmering, sauté the onions, garlic, thyme, and saved mushroom stems on medium-high heat until tender.
- Sauté the walnuts, salt, poultry spice, and paprika until fragrant.
- Remove from the heat and stir in the coconut cream.
- Spoon the mixture into the mushrooms and compact them securely.
- Heat the remaining olive oil in a covered skillet over medium heat.
- Cook the stuffed mushrooms, stuffed side up, for 2 to 3 minutes on medium heat.
- Reduce the heat to low, cover, and simmer for another 10-15 minutes until tender. Garnish with parsley if desired.

Nutritional Information: Per Serving (1 of 12 mushrooms):
- Calories: ~90
- Protein: ~2 g
- Fat: ~8 g
- Saturated Fat: ~2 g
- Carbohydrates: ~3 g

- Fiber: ~1 g
- Sodium: ~150 mg

Grain-Free Crackers

MAKES ABOUT 16 CRACKERS

Ingredients
- 1 cup blanched almond flour
- ¾ cups plus 1 tablespoon tapioca starch
- 2½ tablespoon arrowroot powder
- 1 teaspoon onion powder
- 1 teaspoon iodized sea salt
- ½ teaspoon white pepper
- ⅛ teaspoon xanthan gum
- 1 cup water (approximately)
- ¼ cup toppings of your choice

TOPPING IDEAS:
- Everything: salt, poppy seeds, toasted onion flakes, and black toasted sesame seeds, or Trader
- Joe's "Everything But the Bagel" seasoning
- Caraway seeds and salt
- Fennel seeds and salt
- Rosemary and salt
- Parmigiano-Reggiano cheese

Directions
- Preheat the oven to 350° Fahrenheit. Baking sheets should be lined with silicone nonstick baking sheets (Silpats).
- First, prepare the crackers by combining almond flour, tapioca starch, arrowroot, onion powder, salt, white pepper, and xanthan gum in a medium mixing bowl. Mix thoroughly with a whisk.
- Gradually add the water to the mixture. You want the batter to be thin, like pancake batter. If additional water is required, add it now and stir thoroughly.
- Pour 3 rows of 4 circles of batter onto the baking sheet with a ¼-cup measuring cup or other utensil. Circles should be about 2¾ to 3 inches across. (They will continue to spread slightly after pouring.)
- Sprinkle the appropriate topping on each cracker.
- Bake for 10 minutes at 350°F, then raise the heat to 400°F. (Beginning with a lower temperature prevents crackers from bubbling up in the center, keeping them flat.)
- Bake a further 20 minutes, or until the crackers are brown. Transfer to a cooling rack and, after fully cooled, store in an airtight container for up to 5 days. (Although they lose their crispness after day two, they are still delightful.)

Nutritional Information: Per Cracker (based on 16 crackers):
- Calories: ~40
- Protein: ~1 g Fat: ~3 g
- Saturated Fat: ~0.5 g
- Carbohydrates: ~3 g
- Fiber: ~1 g - Sodium: ~120 mg

Chapter 4

Morning Meals

Carrot Cake Muffins

- **MAKES 12 MUFFINS**

Ingredients
- 1¼ cups blanched almond flour
- 2 tablespoons coconut flour
- ½ teaspoon baking soda
- ⅛ teaspoon salt
- 1½ teaspoons ground cinnamon
- ½ teaspoon ground ginger
- ¼ teaspoon ground nutmeg
- 2 omega-3 or pastured eggs or Vegan Eggs
- ⅓ cup MCT oil or avocado oil
- ⅔ cup unsweetened coconut milk
- ⅓ cup Swerve (erythritol)
- 2 teaspoons vanilla
- 2 large carrots, grated
- ¼ cup chopped walnuts

Directions
- Preheat the oven to 350° Fahrenheit. Line a muffin tray with cupcake liners and leave aside.
- In a large mixing bowl, combine the almond flour, coconut flour, baking soda, salt, cinnamon, ginger, and nutmeg.
- In a small bowl, whisk together the eggs, oil, coconut milk, Swerve, and vanilla.
- Whisk together the wet and dry ingredients, then add the grated carrots and walnuts.
- Fold to merge.
- Pour the mixture into the muffin tin, spreading it evenly between 12 cups.
- Muffins should be baked for 12 to 18 minutes, or until a toothpick inserted in the middle comes out clean. Allow the muffins to cool slightly before serving.
- Muffins will stay fresh in the refrigerator for 5 days or 3 months if stored in an airtight container in the freezer.

Nutritional Information: Per Muffin (based on 12 muffins):
- Calories: ~180
- Protein: ~5 g Fat: ~14 g
- Saturated Fat: ~2 g
- Carbohydrates: ~6 g Fiber: ~3 g
- Sodium: ~150 mg

Caramelized Onion and Gruyère Quiche

SERVES 6

Ingredients
- 1 Plant Paradox Piecrust
- 2 tablespoons extra-virgin olive oil
- 1 medium yellow onion, thinly sliced
- 8 ounces sliced mixed mushrooms, like cremini, oyster, or shiitake
- 2 large pastured or omega-3 eggs or Vegan Eggs
- 2 large egg yolks, or 2 more Vegan Eggs
- ⅔ cup grated Gruyère cheese
- 1¼ cups goat's milk or coconut milk
- ¼ teaspoon iodized sea salt
- ¼ teaspoon white pepper
- Pinch of fresh grated nutmeg (optional)

Directions
- Preheat the oven to 375° Fahrenheit.
- In a medium skillet, heat the oil and sauté the onions slowly, moving constantly, until they are thoroughly browned. Add the sliced mushrooms in the midst of cooking.
- In a large mixing basin, whisk together the eggs and egg yolks. Combine the cheese, goat or coconut milk, salt, white pepper, and nutmeg.
- Place the mushrooms, onions, and cheese in a prebaked pie crust. Distribute equally, then pour the egg mixture on top. Sprinkle with nutmeg, if using.
- Bake for about 30 to 35 minutes, or until lightly browned on top.

Nutritional Information: Per Serving (based on 6 servings):
- Calories: ~300
- Protein: ~12 g
- Fat: ~25 g
- Saturated Fat: ~10 g
- Carbohydrates: ~6 g
- Fiber: ~1 g
- Sodium: ~350 mg

Ralph's Breakfast Scramble

SERVES 1 TO 2

Ingredients
- 1 tablespoon extra-virgin olive oil
- ½ medium onion, diced
- ½ teaspoon iodized sea salt
- ½ teaspoon paprika
- 3 omega-3 or pastured eggs or Vegan Eggs
- ¼ teaspoon pepper
- ½ teaspoon dried basil
- ½ teaspoon Mt. Hood Toasted Onion All Purpose Rub, or ½ teaspoon powdered onion
- ¼ teaspoon cayenne
- ½ ripe avocado, diced

Directions

- In a medium or large skillet, warm the olive oil over low heat.
- Cook the onions, salt, and paprika in a skillet for about 20 minutes, or until lightly caramelized.
- While the onions are caramelizing, in a medium bowl, combine the eggs, a pinch of salt, pepper, basil, Mt. Hood Toasted Onion Rub or onion powder, and cayenne. Mix well.
- Cut the avocado into small squares and add it to the egg mixture, stirring gently.
- In the same skillet as the onions, pour the egg mixture and cook over medium heat. Scramble the eggs and remove from heat when they have reached the desired flavor and texture.

Nutritional Information: Per Serving (based on 2 servings):
- Calories: ~300
- Protein: ~13 g
- Fat: ~25 g
- Saturated Fat: ~4 g
- Carbohydrates: ~10 g
- Fiber: ~7 g
- Sodium: ~350 mg

Cheesy Cauliflower Muffins

MAKES 12 MUFFINS

Ingredients
- 1 tablespoon extra-virgin olive oil
- 3 cups cauliflower rice
- ½ teaspoon iodized sea salt
- ¼ teaspoon garlic powder
- ¼ teaspoon paprika
- ½ teaspoon dried basil
- 3 omega-3 or pastured eggs or Vegan Eggs
- ½ cup grated Parmigiano-Reggiano cheese or nutritional yeast
- ¼ cup cassava flour
- ½ teaspoon aluminum-free baking powder
- Dash of hot sauce (optional)

Directions
- Preheat your oven to 375°F. Line a muffin tray with cupcake liners and leave aside.
- In a sauté pan set over medium-high heat, warm the olive oil. Add the cauliflower rice and sea salt, and simmer for 3 to 5 minutes, stirring constantly.
- Cook for 2 more minutes after adding the garlic powder, paprika, and basil. Allow to cool to room temperature.
- In a large mixing basin, combine the cauliflower, eggs, and cheese or nutritional yeast.
- In a small bowl, combine the cassava flour and baking powder.
- Fold the dry ingredients into the cauliflower mixture, along with the spicy sauce, and then divide into muffin pans.
- Bake for 20-25 minutes, or until the

mixture is no longer wet to the touch. Let cool for at least 5 minutes before serving.

Nutritional Information: Per Muffin (based on 12 muffins):
- Calories: ~120
- Protein: ~6 g
- Fat: ~9 g
- Saturated Fat: ~2 g
- Carbohydrates: ~6 g
- Fiber: ~2 g
- Sodium: ~230 mg

Coconut Macadamia Waffles

SERVES 3 TO 4

Ingredients
- 4 tablespoons MCT oil or melted coconut oil, plus extra for waffle iron
- 4 omega-3 or pastured eggs or Vegan Eggs
- ⅔ cup unsweetened coconut milk
- 5 or 6 drops stevia
- ½ teaspoon vanilla extract
- ½ teaspoon iodized sea salt
- ½ teaspoon aluminum-free baking powder
- ¼ cup coconut flour
- ½ teaspoon cinnamon
- ¼ cup macadamia nuts, finely chopped
- ½ cup coconut cream, to serve

Directions
- Preheat your waffle iron according to the manufacturer's directions.
- In a large bowl, combine the oil, eggs, coconut milk, stevia, and vanilla essence.
- Add the dry ingredients to the wet and whisk until well blended.
- Fold in the macadamia nuts.
- Coat the waffle iron with MCT or coconut oil, then cook as directed by your model, using about one-third of a cup batter each 4-inch square waffle.
- Garnish with coconut cream before serving.

Nutritional Information: Per Waffle (based on 4 servings)
- Calories: ~220
- Protein: ~5 g
- Fat: ~18 g
- Saturated Fat: ~10 g
- Carbohydrates: ~6 g
- Fiber: ~3 g
- Sugar: ~1 g
- Sodium: ~150 mg

Chocolate Chip Mini-Pancakes

SERVES 3 TO 4 (MAKES 12 TO 14 MINI-PANCAKES)

Ingredients
- 6 omega-3 or pastured eggs or VeganEggs
- 1½ cups water

- 2 teaspoons almond extract
- 1 cup coconut flour
- ½ cup tapioca starch
- ½ cup arrowroot starch
- 2 tablespoons monk-fruit sweetener or 1 packet stevia
- 1 teaspoon baking powder
- 1 teaspoon baking soda
- ¼ teaspoon iodized sea salt
- 1 cup 85 to 90 percent cacao chocolate, finely chopped
- 1 tablespoon ghee or coconut oil

Directions

- Preheat the oven to 200°F (to keep cooked pancakes warm).
- In a large mixing basin, whisk together the eggs, water, and almond essence.
- Combine the coconut flour, tapioca starch, arrowroot starch, monk fruit sweetener, baking powder, baking soda, and salt.
- Mix until the batter is smooth. Add the finely chopped chocolate and combine well.
- Heat your griddle or ceramic nonstick pan to medium heat, then add the ghee or coconut oil.
- For 3-inch pancakes, use slightly less than a quarter cup of batter.
- When bubbles develop, turn the pancakes and cook for another 2-3 minutes, or until golden brown.
- Serve immediately or reheat in the oven. If you want to serve them later or freeze them, place them in a toaster oven to warm up. (Allow frozen pancakes to defrost for about an hour before toasting.)

Nutritional Info (per pancake):
- Calories: ~120
- Protein: ~5g
- Fat: ~9g
- Carbs: ~8g
- Fiber: ~3g
- Sugar: ~1g

Broccoli Cheddar Quiche

SERVES 8

Ingredients

FOR THE CRUST (or see Plant Paradox Piecrust)
- 1¼ cups coconut flour
- ½ cup toasted macadamia nuts, finely chopped
- 1 cup coconut oil
- 1 omega-3 or pastured egg or Vegan Egg

FOR THE FILLING
- 2 cups broccoli florets, cut into small pieces
- 5 omega-3 or pastured eggs or Vegan Eggs
- ⅔ cup unsweetened coconut cream
- ¼ teaspoon nutmeg
- 1 teaspoon iodized sea salt

- 1 cup shredded goat's milk cheddar cheese or ½ cup nutritional yeast

Directions
- Preheat the oven to 400° Fahrenheit. Coat an 8-inch pie tin in olive oil.
- First, prepare the crust by pulsing the coconut flour, macadamia nuts, coconut oil, and egg in a food processor until the dough comes together. If the mixture is too dry, add water one teaspoon at a time until it becomes cohesive. The mixture will be slightly crumbly, akin to a graham cracker crust.
- Take the dough out of the food processor, wrap it in plastic wrap, and put it in the refrigerator for an hour.
- Press the dough into the pie tin with your fingertips and bake for 10 minutes. Set aside to cool. Reduce the oven temperature to 350°F.
- Steam broccoli for 2-3 minutes, then drain and set aside.
- Combine the eggs, coconut cream, nutmeg, and salt, and stir thoroughly.
- Put the crust on a sheet tray in case it overflows while baking.
- Sprinkle the bottom of the crust with cheddar cheese or nutritional yeast, followed by the broccoli.
- Cover with the egg mixture and bake for 35 to 40 minutes at 350°F. Let cool for a few minutes before serving.

Nutritional Information (per serving):
- Calories: ~250
- Protein: ~7g
- Fat: ~21g
- Carbs: ~8g
- Fiber: ~3g
- Sugar: ~2g

Pesto-Baked Eggs

SERVES 4

Ingredients
- 5 teaspoons extra-virgin olive oil
- 2 cups thinly sliced kale or Swiss chard
- 2 cloves garlic, minced
- ½ teaspoon iodized sea salt
- 4 omega-3 or pastured eggs or Vegan Eggs
- 4 tablespoons Classic Basil Pesto

Directions
- Preheat the oven to 350° Fahrenheit. Pour one teaspoon olive oil into each of four 6- to 8-ounce ramekins.
- Heat the final teaspoon of oil in a large sauté pan. Cook for about 3 minutes, stirring in the kale or chard, garlic, and sea salt.
- Divide the garlic into the ramekins, and then crack one egg into each.
- Top with pesto and bake for 10-15 minutes, or until the egg is set.

Nutritional Information (per serving):
- Calories: ~180

- Protein: ~7g
- Fat: ~15g
- Carbs: ~3g
- Fiber: ~1g
- Sugar: ~1g

"Pumpkin" Spice Sweet Potato Pancakes

SERVES 1 TO 2

Ingredients

- 1 small sweet potato, baked, peeled, and mashed (approximately ½ cup)
- 4 to 5 drops stevia
- 2 teaspoons unsweetened coconut milk
- 2 omega-3 or pastured eggs or Vegan Eggs
- ½ teaspoon aluminum-free baking powder
- 3 tablespoons blanched almond flour
- ¼ teaspoon cinnamon
- ¼ teaspoon ground nutmeg
- ⅛ teaspoon ground cloves
- ¼ teaspoon ground ginger
- Zest of 1 orange
- French or Italian grass-fed butter (such as Trader Joe's Cultured French Butter, President, or Beurre D'Insigny), ghee, or avocado oil for cooking and serving

Directions

- Whisk the sweet potato, stevia, coconut milk, and eggs together until completely incorporated.
- Combine the baking powder, almond flour, spices, and orange zest into the mixture.
- Heat a skillet over medium-high heat and add the butter. When it's melted, add one-third of a cup pancake batter to the skillet and cook for 3 to 4 minutes. With a spatula, flip and cook for a further 3 to 4 minutes, or until golden brown.
- Continue with the remaining batter and serve.

Nutritional Information (per serving):
- Calories: ~200
- Protein: ~8g
- Fat: ~11g
- Carbs: ~17g
- Fiber: ~3g
- Sugar: ~4g

"Bacon"-and-Egg Breakfast Salad

SERVES 2

Ingredients

- Juice of 1 lemon
- ¼ cup red wine vinegar
- ½ cup extra-virgin olive oil
- ½ teaspoon Dijon mustard
- 2 cups baby spinach
- 2 cups shredded kale, stems removed

- 2 hard boiled eggs, chopped
- 3 ounces prosciutto, finely chopped, or vegan bacon pieces
- ½ cup broccoli slaw (shredded broccoli stalks sold in bags in the produce section)
- ½ avocado, diced
- ¼ cup unsweetened dried cranberries

Directions
- In a large mixing bowl, combine the lemon juice, vinegar, olive oil, and mustard.
- Toss in the spinach and kale until well combined.
- Garnish with eggs, prosciutto or vegan bacon, broccoli slaw, avocado, and dried cranberries. Enjoy immediately.

Nutritional Information (per serving):
- Calories: ~350
- Protein: ~15g
- Fat: ~28g
- Carbs: ~13g
- Fiber: ~5g
- Sugar: ~6g

Chapter 5

Soups and Stews

Chicken and Vegetable (Miracle) Rice Soup

SERVES 4

Ingredients

- ¼ cup extra-virgin olive oil
- 1 onion, diced
- 3 celery stalks, diced
- 2 cloves garlic, minced
- 2 cups mushrooms, diced
- 1 teaspoon dried sage
- 1 teaspoon fresh thyme
- ½ teaspoon fresh rosemary
- ½ teaspoon black pepper
- Zest of 1 lemon
- Juice of 1 lemon
- 1 teaspoon iodized sea salt
- 1 cup diced cooked pasture-raised chicken or Quorn crumbles
- 4 cups Bone Broth or organic, low-sodium chicken or vegetable broth
- 2 packages Miracle Rice

Directions

- Warm the olive oil in a large soup pot over medium-high heat. Cook the onion and celery until soft and transparent, about 5 or 6 minutes.
- Cook the garlic and mushrooms, together with the sage, thyme, rosemary, pepper, lemon zest, lemon juice, and salt, stirring frequently, until soft, about 3 to 5 minutes.
- Add the chicken (or Quorn) and stock, then decrease the heat to low and cook for 15 to 20 minutes. Before serving, add the Miracle Rice and cook for 1 to 2 minutes, or until thoroughly heated.

Nutritional Information (per serving):
- Calories: ~180
- Protein: ~10g
- Fat: ~12g
- Carbs: ~7g
- Fiber: ~2g
- Sugar: ~3g

Creamy Sweet Potato Soup

SERVES 4 TO 6

Ingredients
- 2 tablespoons extra-virgin olive oil
- 1 small onion, diced
- 3 celery stalks, diced
- 3 to 4 sweet potatoes (about 2 pounds), peeled and cut into 1-inch cubes
- 2 cloves garlic, chopped
- 1 to 2 teaspoons iodized sea salt
- 1 teaspoon freshly ground black pepper
- 1 teaspoon paprika
- 1 teaspoon fresh thyme
- ½ teaspoon cinnamon
- 4 cups chicken stock or Vegetable Stock
- Parmesan cheese, to garnish (optional)
- Extra fresh ground black pepper, to taste

Directions
- The olive oil should be heated in a large soup pot over medium-high heat. Sauté the onions and celery until they are soft and transparent.
- Sauté the sweet potatoes, garlic, sea salt, pepper, paprika, thyme, and cinnamon until the thyme is aromatic and the sweet potatoes start to soften around the edges.
- Put the stock in and turn the heat down to low. Cover and boil for 30 minutes, or until the sweet potatoes are falling apart.
- Transfer the contents to a high-speed blender (or immersion blender) and puree until smooth.
- Garnish with cheese (if desired) and black pepper.

Nutritional Information (per serving, serves 6):
- Calories: ~160
- Protein: ~2g
- Fat: ~6g
- Carbs: ~25g
- Fiber: ~4g
- Sugar: ~6g

Dr. G's Bean Chili

SERVES 4

Ingredients
- ¼ cup olive oil
- 1 large onion, chopped
- 5 cloves garlic, minced
- 1 red bell pepper, peeled, seeded, and chopped
- 1 poblano pepper, peeled, seeded, and chopped
- 1 jalapeño pepper, peeled, seeded, and diced
- 1 cup dried red beans, picked over, rinsed, and soaked 24–48 hours in 2 changes of water
- 1 cup dried black beans, picked over, rinsed, and soaked in 2 changes of water
- 1 cup dried lentils, picked over, and soaked in 2 changes of water

- 5 cups peeled, seeded, and minced tomatoes (about 7 tomatoes)
- 3 cups water or vegetable broth
- 2 tablespoons chili powder
- 1 tablespoon chipotle puree (optional, but recommended)
- 1 tablespoon ground cumin
- 1 teaspoon iodized sea salt, more to taste
- ½ cup shredded goat's milk cheddar, to serve (optional)
- 1 cup diced cilantro, to serve (optional)

Directions
- Heat the olive oil in a big pot (or in a pressure cooker on sauté mode) over medium-high heat.
- Sauté the onions, garlic, and peppers until fragrant, about 5 to 7 minutes, before transferring to the pressure cooker.
- Stir in the beans, lentils, tomatoes, broth or water, spices (include chipotle puree if wanted), and salt to mix.
- Cook for roughly 10 minutes on high pressure, following your pressure cooker's directions.
- Allow the pressure cooker to depressurize, then remove from heat, mix, and serve. If desired, sprinkle with cheddar or cilantro.

Nutritional Information (per serving, serves 4):
- Calories: ~320
- Protein: ~14g
- Fat: ~12g
- Carbs: ~42g
- Fiber: ~12g
- Sugar: ~6g

Leek and Cauliflower Soup

SERVES 4 TO 6

Ingredients
- 3 tablespoons extra-virgin olive oil
- 1 pound leeks, cleaned and chopped
- 2 celery stalks, diced
- 3 cloves garlic, minced
- 1 large head of cauliflower, cut into 2-inch florets
- ½ teaspoon fresh nutmeg
- 1 teaspoon fine iodized sea salt, or more, to taste
- 2 teaspoons coarse black pepper
- 2 quarts salt-free chicken stock or Vegetable Stock
- ¼ cup grated Parmesan (optional, but delicious)
- 1 bay leaf
- Finely chopped chives or thyme, to garnish

Directions
- The olive oil should be heated in a large soup pot over medium-high heat. Sauté the leeks, celery, garlic, and cauliflower, along with the nutmeg, salt, and pepper, over

- medium heat, stirring often until the leeks wilt.
- Cook, covered, for 35 to 45 minutes until the cauliflower is extremely soft.
- Remove the bay leaf and process with an immersion stick blender or in a conventional blender until smooth (working in stages to avoid overfilling).
- Once blended, return the soup to the heat and simmer for another 10 to 15 minutes.
- Garnish with chopped herbs and additional Parmesan, if preferred.

Nutritional Information (per serving, serves 4-6):
- Calories: ~130
- Protein: ~4g
- Fat: ~9g
- Carbs: ~10g
- Fiber: ~3g
- Sugar: ~3g

Lemon, Kale, and Chicken Soup

SERVES 4 TO 6

Ingredients
- 3 tablespoons extra-virgin olive oil
- 1 medium onion, finely diced
- 4 cloves garlic, minced
- 2 celery stalks, minced
- Freshly ground black pepper, to taste
- Iodized sea salt, to taste
- 1 cup cooked pastured chicken (white or dark meat—perfect for using up whatever leftover chicken you have on hand), cubed or shredded, or 1 cup Quorn crumbles
- ½ teaspoon Dijon mustard
- 2 bunches kale, cut into 1-inch pieces
- Zest of 1 lemon
- 5 cups Chicken Bone Broth or Vegetable Stock
- 1 teaspoon balsamic vinegar 2 tablespoons fresh lemon juice
- Freshly grated Parmigiano Reggiano, for serving (optional)

Directions
- In a large soup pot, heat the olive oil over medium heat. Combine the onion, garlic, and celery with the black pepper and a little amount of sea salt. Sauté until the onion and celery are extremely soft.
- Sauté the chicken or Quorn, mustard, kale, and lemon zest for a further 5 minutes.
- Reduce the heat and mix in the stock, balsamic vinegar, and lemon juice. Cover and cook for 35 minutes.
- Ladle into dishes and garnish with fresh black pepper and cheese, if preferred.

Nutritional Information (per serving, serves 4-6):

- Calories: ~160
- Protein: ~14g
- Fat: ~8g
- Carbs: ~10g
- Fiber: ~2g
- Sugar: ~2g

"Cream" of Mushroom Soup

SERVES 8

Ingredients
- 3 tablespoons extra-virgin olive oil
- 2 pounds mushrooms, finely diced
- 1 teaspoon fresh thyme
- Zest of 1 lemon
- 1 onion, diced
- 2 cloves garlic, minced
- 2 celery stalks, diced
- 1 large head cauliflower, outer leaves removed, coarsely chopped
- 1½ teaspoons iodized sea salt
- ½ teaspoon black pepper
- ½ teaspoon onion powder
- 1 teaspoon Dijon mustard
- 4 cups Bone Broth or organic, low-sodium chicken or vegetable broth
- 1 cup unsweetened coconut cream

Directions
- In a large soup pot, warm 2 tablespoons olive oil over medium heat. Cook the mushrooms till golden brown and soft, then add the thyme and lemon and cook for another 2 minutes, or until extremely fragrant.
- Set half of the mushrooms aside and leave the rest in the pot. Cook the remaining olive oil, onion, garlic, and celery until soft.
- Place the cauliflower in the pot, along with the salt, pepper, onion powder, and mustard.
- Sauté until aromatic, then add broth. Cook until the cauliflower is soft, about 5 to 7 minutes, then purée in a blender.
- When the soup is smooth, add the reserved mushrooms and coconut cream. Stir to blend, then serve.

Nutritional Information (per serving, serves 8):
- Calories: ~110
- Protein: ~4g
- Fat: ~6g
- Carbs: ~9g
- Fiber: ~2g
- Sugar: ~3g

Mushroom Coconut Curry

SERVES 8

Ingredients
- 1 tablespoon coconut oil
- 1 small white onion, diced
- 2 cloves garlic, pressed or minced
- 1 tablespoon minced fresh ginger

- 2 cups broccoli slaw (the packaged, shredded broccoli stalks available in the produce section of most grocery stores)
- 2 cups sliced brown mushrooms
- 2 tablespoons Thai red curry paste
- 1 14-ounce can unsweetened coconut milk
- ½ cup water or broth
- 1½ cups packed thinly sliced kale
- 5 to 6 drops stevia
- 1 tablespoon fish sauce or coconut aminos
- Juice of 1 lime
- 1 small handful basil or cilantro, chopped

Directions

- In a big soup pot, heat the oil over medium-high heat. Cook the onion until transparent, then add the garlic and ginger.
- After the ginger and garlic are aromatic, add the broccoli slaw and mushrooms. Cook over medium-high heat for 4 to 6 minutes, or until the mushrooms are cooked.
- Stir in the curry paste until thoroughly blended. Cook for 1–2 minutes, until very fragrant.
- Reduce the heat to low and stir in the coconut milk, water or broth, kale, stevia, and fish sauce. Allow to simmer for 20 minutes before turning off the heat. Add the lime juice, basil, or cilantro, and serve.

Nutritional Info (Per Serving):
- Calories: ~110
- Protein: ~3 g
- Carbs: ~7 g (Fiber: ~2 g)
- Fat: ~9 g (Sat. Fat: ~7 g)
- Sodium: ~300-400 mg

Not-Quite-French Onion Soup

SERVES 6 TO 8

Ingredients
- ¼ cup extra-virgin olive oil
- 5 large sweet onions (like Maui or Vidalia), thinly sliced
- 2 tablespoons red wine vinegar
- 6 cloves garlic, thinly sliced
- 2 bay leaves
- 1 teaspoon chopped fresh thyme
- ½ teaspoon ground black pepper
- 6 cups Bone Broth or Vegetable Stock or water, or a combination of the three
- Iodized sea salt, to taste
- Grated Gruyère or Parmesan cheese, to taste, for serving

Directions
- Heat the olive oil on a low heat. Cook the onions, turning constantly, until dark brown and caramelized, about 15 minutes.
- Reduce the heat to low and stir in the vinegar and garlic. Cook, stirring regularly, until the garlic is aromatic,

- about 2 minutes.
- Add the bay leaves, thyme, pepper, and broth or stock, and simmer for 15 to 20 minutes, covered. Uncover and cook for a further 10 to 15 minutes before removing from heat. Remove the bay leaves and sprinkle with salt to taste.
- Pour the soup into ramekins or small bowls and garnish with shredded cheese. If the heat from the soup is insufficient to melt the cheese, set the oven-safe bowls on a sheet pan and broil for 30 seconds to 1 minute.

Nutritional Info (Per Serving):
- Calories: ~150
- Protein: ~3 g
- Carbs: ~15 g (Fiber: ~2 g)
- Fat: ~10 g (Sat. Fat: ~2 g)
- Sodium: ~300-400 mg (varies with broth and cheese)

Beef and Mushroom Stew

SERVES 6 TO 8

Ingredients
- 1 pound pastured sirloin, cubed, or 16 ounces cubed tempeh
- 2 tablespoons cassava flour
- ¼ cup extra-virgin olive oil
- 1 large onion, diced
- 3 celery stalks, minced
- 3 cloves garlic, minced
- 1 pound mushrooms, sliced
- 1 teaspoon iodized sea salt
- 1 tablespoon fresh thyme leaves
- 1 cup red wine
- 2 cups Bone Broth or vegetable broth
- 1 tablespoon red wine vinegar

Directions
- In a mixing basin, combine the cassava flour and sirloin (or tempeh) until evenly covered.
- In a large soup pot, heat the olive oil over medium heat.
- Cook the sirloin or tempeh on all sides until golden brown.
- Add the mushrooms, celery, onion, and garlic. Cook, turning frequently, until the garlic is fragrant and the veggies are soft, about 4 to 6 minutes.
- Sauté for another minute, or until aromatic, with the sea salt and thyme.
- Deglaze the pot with the wine, broth, and vinegar, scraping the bottom of the pan to remove any brown, cooked-on deliciousness.
- Reduce the heat to low and cook for 45 minutes to an hour, adding water as required, until the beef is very soft.
- Serve with mashed cauliflower or sweet potatoes.

Nutritional Info (Per Serving):

- Calories: ~250
- Protein: ~20 g (with sirloin; ~10 g with tempeh)
- Carbs: ~10 g (Fiber: ~2 g)
- Fat: ~14 g (Sat. Fat: ~2 g)
- Sodium: ~400 mg (varies with broth and added salt)

Sweet Potato and Spinach Curry

SERVES 2 TO 4

Ingredients
- 3 to 4 teaspoons avocado oil
- 1⅓ teaspoon mustard seeds
- ⅓ teaspoon cumin seeds
- 1 green cardamom pod
- 3 whole cloves
- 3 minced garlic cloves
- 1 red onion, minced
- 1 medium sweet potato, peeled and diced
- ½ teaspoon turmeric
- ⅓ teaspoon cinnamon powder
- 1 teaspoon crushed black pepper
- 2 cups coconut milk or water
- 2 cups baby spinach
- Iodized sea salt, to taste

Directions
- In a big stainless steel skillet, heat 1 teaspoon of avocado oil over low heat. Then, add the mustard and cumin seeds and roast for 20 seconds.
- Roast the cardamom and cloves together for 1 minute, stirring often.
- Remove from heat and process in a spice grinder until powdered.
- Add the remaining oil to the pan, along with the garlic and onions.
- Sauté the garlic and onion over medium heat for 2 to 4 minutes, or until golden brown.
- Add the black pepper, turmeric, and cinnamon, as well as the powdered spices you toasted in steps 1 and 2, and continue to sauté for 3 to 4 minutes after adding the sweet potato.
- Add the spinach and coconut milk or water, and simmer for 15 to 20 minutes, or until the sweet potatoes are very soft.
- Season to taste with salt before serving.

Nutritional Info (Per Serving):
- Calories: ~220
- Protein: ~3 g
- Carbs: ~30 g (Fiber: ~6 g)
- Fat: ~12 g (Sat. Fat: ~9 g from coconut milk)
- Sodium: ~200-300 mg (varies with salt and coconut milk)

Chapter 6

Noodles and Bowls

Banh Mi Bowl

SERVES 1

Ingredients

DRESSING
- ¼ avocado
- ¼ cup cilantro
- Juice of 1 lime
- 1 teaspoon garlic chili sauce or Sriracha
- 1 teaspoon sesame oil
- 1 teaspoon rice wine vinegar

BOWL
- 1 tablespoon toasted sesame oil
- 2 ounces pasture-raised chicken, diced, or ½ cup Quorn crumbles
- ½ teaspoon yacón syrup
- ½ teaspoon fish sauce or coconut aminos
- ½ teaspoon rice wine vinegar
- 2 cups mixed salad greens
- ¼ cup pickled daikon
- ¼ cup pickled red onions
- ¼ cup pickled carrots
- 1 omega-3 or pastured egg, soft-boiled and peeled

Directions
- In a blender, combine all of the dressing ingredients and pulse until smooth. Set aside.
- Heat the sesame oil in a sauté pan over medium heat until it is warm and aromatic. Saute the Quorn or chicken for 3 to 4 minutes, stirring occasionally.
- Mix in the yacón syrup, fish sauce or coconut aminos, and rice wine vinegar, then reduce the heat to low. Continue heating until the meat is done and the mixture is well browned.
- Before putting the salad leaves in the serving bowl, toss them with the dressing.
- Place the pork, daikon, red onion, carrots, and egg on top of the leaves. Serve, and enjoy!

Nutritional Info (Per Serving):
- Calories: ~300
- Protein: ~18 g

- Carbs: ~14 g (Fiber: ~4 g)
- Fat: ~20 g (Sat. Fat: ~4 g)
- Sodium: ~450-600 mg (varies with fish sauce and pickled vegetables)

Shrimp Poke Bowl

SERVES 1

Ingredients

- 1 tablespoon rice wine vinegar
- 1 tablespoon coconut aminos
- 2 tablespoon avocado mayonnaise
- 1 teaspoon sesame seeds
- 1 to 2 drops stevia
- 1 tablespoon diced dried seaweed (nori), crumbled
- 1 tablespoon sesame oil
- 1 teaspoon fresh minced ginger
- 1 clove garlic, minced
- 3 ounces wild shrimp, deveined, shelled (or leave shells on if you like their lectin-fighting abilities!), and chopped, or hearts of palm
- 1 cup steamed cauliflower rice
- ¼ avocado
- ¼ cup seaweed salad (optional, available at many Japanese markets or in the sushi bar section at your local store)
- Sriracha or other hot sauce (optional)

Directions

- Mix together the rice vinegar, coconut aminos, mayonnaise, sesame seeds, stevia, and seaweed. Set aside.
- In a medium-sized skillet, heat the sesame oil. Combine ginger, garlic, and shrimp. Cook for 2 to 3 minutes, tossing periodically, until the shrimp are fully cooked.
- Toss the shrimp with the sauce.
- If using, top with the avocado and seaweed salad and serve over cauliflower rice. Drizzle with Sriracha if preferred and serve.

Nutritional Info (Per Serving):

- Calories: ~280
- Protein: ~20 g
- Carbs: ~8 g (Fiber: ~4 g)
- Fat: ~18 g (Sat. Fat: ~3 g)
- Sodium: ~600-800 mg (varies with coconut aminos and seaweed salad)

Egg Roll in a Bowl

SERVES 2 TO 4

Ingredients

- 2 tablespoons sesame oil
- 3 cloves garlic, minced
- 1 yellow onion, diced
- 4 green onions, thinly sliced
- 1 tablespoon fresh ginger, minced
- 1 bag Quorn grounds or 1 cup wild-caught shrimp
- Iodized sea salt and black pepper, to taste
- 1 tablespoon garlic chili sauce or Sriracha (use less or more, to taste)
- 3 cups shredded cabbage
- 2 cups broccoli slaw (shredded

- broccoli stalks sold packaged in the produce section)
- 3 tablespoons coconut aminos
- 1 tablespoon rice wine vinegar
- 2 tablespoons toasted sesame seeds

Directions
- In a big wok or sauté pan, heat the sesame oil over medium-high heat.
- Cook the garlic, onion, green onion, and ginger until they are tender and fragrant.
- Stir in the Quorn grinds or shrimp, salt, pepper, and garlic chili sauce (if using), and cook until the Quorn is warmed through or the shrimp is light pink.
- Toss the cabbage, broccoli slaw, coconut aminos, rice vinegar, and sesame seeds into the wok, then simmer until the cabbage is soft.
- Serve immediately.

Nutritional Info (Per Serving):
- Calories: ~200
- Protein: ~15 g
- Carbs: ~10 g (Fiber: ~4 g)
- Fat: ~12 g (Sat. Fat: ~2 g)
- Sodium: ~500-700 mg (varies with coconut aminos and garlic chili sauce)

Sorghum Bowl

SERVES 1

Ingredients

- 1 tablespoon olive oil
- ½ small yellow onion, minced
- 1 clove garlic, minced
- ½ cup Quorn crumbles
- 1 cup cooked sorghum
- ¼ cup pickled carrots
- ¼ cup pickled beets
- ¼ cup pickled onions
- ¼ cup pickled radishes*
- ½ avocado, diced

Directions
- In a medium pan set over medium-high heat, heat the olive oil.
- Sauté the onion for 2-3 minutes, or until tender. Sauté the garlic for another minute, until aromatic.
- Cook the Quorn crumbles and sorghum, stirring frequently, until the flavors combine.
- Place in a serving bowl and top with the pickled veggies and avocado. Serve immediately.

Nutritional Info (Per Serving):
- Calories: ~350
- Protein: ~12 g
- Carbs: ~40 g (Fiber: ~8 g)
- Fat: ~14 g (Sat. Fat: ~2 g)
- Sodium: ~600-800 mg (varies with pickled veggies)

Baby Zucchini Noodles with Creamy Avocado Sauce

SERVES 2 TO 3

Ingredients
- 1 tablespoon avocado oil
- 4 ounces boneless, skinless chicken breast (pastured), cut into strips (optional)
- ¼ teaspoon iodized sea salt
- ¼ teaspoon freshly cracked black pepper
- 1 large endive, shredded
- 12 fresh asparagus spears, cut into 2- to 3-inch pieces
- 8 baby zucchinis, spiralized,* set aside
- ¼ cup blanched almonds, chopped (slivered almonds work as well)

FOR THE AVOCADO SAUCE
- 1 large ripe avocado
- ½ cup full-fat coconut milk
- ½ cup water
- Juice of 1 lemon
- ½ teaspoon salt
- ¼ teaspoon freshly cracked black pepper
- 1 teaspoon fresh thyme

Directions
- Place the chicken in the avocado oil over medium-high heat (or on to step 2 if you are not using chicken). Season with salt and pepper and sauté for 5 to 6 minutes, or until well cooked.
- Continue heating until the endive and asparagus are tender, about 3 to 4 minutes.
- While the chicken and vegetables cook, combine all of the avocado sauce ingredients in a food processor with an S-blade and process until smooth and creamy.
- Combine the reserved zucchini with the chicken (if using) and veggies, mixing thoroughly. The heat alone will cook and soften the zucchini.
- Stir in the avocado sauce, then top with the chopped almonds and serve.

Nutritional Info (Per Serving):
- Calories: ~320
- Protein: ~18 g (with chicken; ~5 g without)
- Carbs: ~12 g (Fiber: ~6 g)
- Fat: ~24 g (Sat. Fat: ~6 g)
- Sodium: ~450 mg

Creamy Shrimp and Kale Spaghetti

SERVES 2

Ingredients
- ¼ cup extra-virgin olive oil

- 1 brown onion, thinly sliced
- 3 cloves garlic, thinly sliced
- 6 ounces wild-caught shrimp, deveined (optional)
- 2 cups thinly sliced kale
- 1 cup unsweetened coconut cream
- Juice of 1 lemon
- ¼ cup grated Parmigiano-Reggiano or 2 tablespoons nutritional yeast

FOR THE MIRACLE NOODLES, COOKED THE GUNDRY WAY
- 1 package Miracle Noodles spaghetti
- Iodized sea salt, to taste.

Directions
- In a large skillet, heat the olive oil over medium heat.
- Add the onion and sauté for 3 to 4 minutes, or until soft and transparent.
- Cook for an additional 2 minutes, until the shrimp are pink and the garlic is aromatic.
- Turn the heat down to low and add the greens, coconut cream, and lemon. Cook until the kale wilts, then add the Parmigiano or yeast.
- Cook for 3–4 minutes before adding the Miracle Noodles. Cook for an additional 2 minutes, then serve.

FOR THE MIRACLE NOODLES, COOKED THE GUNDRY WAY
- Heat a kettle of salted water to a boil.
- Take the noodles out of the package and rinse them under cold running water for 2-3 minutes.
- Add the noodles to the boiling water and cook for 2-3 minutes.
- Transfer to a dry pan and simmer over medium-low heat, stirring until the noodles are dry.

Not Bad Pad Thai

SERVES 2

Ingredients
- 2 tablespoons olive oil
- 1 tablespoon sesame oil
- 2 garlic cloves
- 6 ounces wild shrimp, shells off (optional)
- ½ cup broccoli slaw (optional)
- 1 omega-3 or pastured egg or VeganEgg
- ½ cup basil leaves, chopped
- One 8-ounce package fettuccine-style Miracle Noodles
- Juice of 2 limes
- 4 tablespoons chopped dry roasted macadamia nuts
- 1 to 2 tablespoons fish sauce or coconut aminos
- 1 tablespoon unsweetened, unseasoned rice vinegar
- Pinch of stevia
- 1 teaspoon paprika

Directions
- The oils should be heated in a big skillet over high heat, but not so hot that they smoke.

- Stir in the garlic momentarily, then add the shrimp and broccoli slaw (if using) and cook for another minute.
- Stir in the egg for one further minute, or until cooked.
- Stir-fry for approximately three more minutes, or until the shrimp are opaque, after adding the basil, noodles, lime juice, macadamia nuts, fish sauce or coconut aminos, rice vinegar, paprika, and stevia. Serve soon after removing from heat.

Nutritional Info (Per Serving):
- Calories: ~320
- Protein: ~18 g
- Carbs: ~10 g (Fiber: ~3 g)
- Fat: ~25 g (Sat. Fat: ~4 g)
- Sodium: ~600-800 mg (varies with fish sauce and added salt)

Truffled Mushroom Mac and Cheese

SERVES 1

Ingredients

FOR THE CHEESE SAUCE
- 1 cup raw macadamia nuts, soaked for 8 hours or overnight
- ¾ cup water
- Juice from ½ lemon
- ¼ cup nutritional yeast
- 1 teaspoon iodized sea salt
- ½ teaspoon smoked paprika
- ⅛ teaspoon powdered mustard
- ½ clove garlic
- Pinch of black pepper

FOR THE MAC AND CHEESE
- 1 package ziti-style Miracle Noodles or fettucine, cut into small pieces
- 2 teaspoons buffalo ghee or avocado oil
- 2 large oyster mushrooms, roughly chopped
- ¼ cup cheese sauce
- 1 handful fresh spinach
- Iodized sea salt and black pepper to taste
- Nutritional yeast to sprinkle
- ½ teaspoon truffle oil

Directions
- First, prepare the cheese sauce: Put all the ingredients in the work bowl of a food processor with an S-blade or in a high-speed blender like a Vitamix or Blendtec.
- Blend at high speed until smooth. If the mixture becomes too thick, add more water, one tablespoon at a time.
- Make the Miracle Noodle ziti the Gundry way. Set aside.
- Saute the oyster mushrooms in a small-to-sized saucepan over medium heat with the buffalo ghee or avocado oil.
- Once tender, add the noodles, cheese sauce, and spinach, and cook over medium-low heat until the spinach is wilted.

- Stir in the truffle oil, nutritional yeast, salt, and pepper until well combined.

Nutritional Info (Per Serving):
- Calories: ~420
- Protein: ~12 g
- Carbs: ~15 g (Fiber: ~7 g)
- Fat: ~35 g (Sat. Fat: ~6 g)
- Sodium: ~550 mg

Fettuccine with Red Capsicum and Carrot

SERVES 4

Ingredients
- 375g fettuccine
- 2 tablespoons slivered almonds
- 3 tablespoons extra-virgin olive oil
- 2 red capsicums, seeded and sliced
- 1 large carrot, grated
- 2 cloves garlic, peeled
- 2–3 cups fresh basil leaves
- 2 tablespoons lemon juice

Directions
- Cook the fettuccine as directed on the package, being careful not to overcook it. Drain well.
- While the fettuccine cooks, toast the almonds in a dry frying pan, stirring frequently to prevent them from burning. When golden brown, place them on a platter.
- In the same pan, heat 1 tablespoon of oil and gently sauté the capsicum for around 5 minutes, stirring frequently.
- Grate the carrot with a food processor. Change to a chopping blade and combine the garlic, basil, lemon juice, remaining oil, and capsicum. Blend, but not too much that the texture is lost. Add the almonds and stir.
- Toss the fettuccine with the capsicum mixture. Serve immediately in hot bowls.

Nutritional Info (Per Serving):
- Calories: ~370
- Protein: ~10 g
- Carbs: ~45 g (Fiber: 11 g)
- Fat: ~15 g (Sat. Fat: 2.5 g)
- Sodium: ~30 mg (may vary based on added salt)

Spaghetti with Chicken and Lemon

SERVES 4

Ingredients
- 375g spaghetti
- 1 tablespoon extra-virgin olive oil
- 1 medium onion, sliced
- 1–2 cloves garlic, peeled and crushed
- 250g skinless chicken breast fillet, sliced
- 2 teaspoons finely grated lemon zest
- juice of 1 lemon

- 2 tablespoons chopped fresh basil or flat-leaf parsley or dill
- 2 tablespoons balsamic vinegar

Directions
- Cook the spaghetti according to the package directions, taking care not to overcook. Drain well.
- While the spaghetti is boiling, heat the olive oil in a frying pan or wok and saute the onion, garlic, and chicken. Stir-fry the chicken for 5 minutes, or until it is golden but not dry. Combine lemon zest, juice, basil, and balsamic vinegar.
- Serve spaghetti in hot dishes, topped with the chicken mixture.

Nutritional Highlights (Approx. Per Serving):
- Calories: ~380
- Protein: ~25 g
- Carbohydrates: ~45 g (Fiber: 6 g)
- Fat: ~8 g (Sat. Fat: 1.5 g)
- Sodium: ~50 mg (adjust based on added salt).

Chapter 7

Main Dishes

Superfood Salad

SERVES 1

Ingredients

- 2 cups baby kale and arugula
- ¼ cup artichoke hearts, frozen and thawed, minced (canned will work in a pinch, just make sure they have no sugar added, and rinse them well before using)
- ½ cup broccoli slaw
- ¼ cup raw red beets, shredded
- ¼ cup radishes, sliced
- 2 tablespoons Classic Balsamic Vinaigrette
- ¼ cup pomegranate seeds (if in season, September through January)
- ½ avocado, diced
- 1 omega-3 or pastured egg, hard-boiled and crumbled (optional)

Directions

- Fill a large salad bowl with the greens, artichoke hearts, broccoli slaw, beets, radishes, and vinaigrette. Toss with salad tongs or clean hands until fully combined.
- Transfer to a platter and decorate with pomegranate seeds, avocado, and egg, if desired.

Nutritional Information Per Serving

- Calories: ~350-400
- Protein: ~9-10g
- Carbs: ~35g
- Fiber: ~12g
- Fat: ~25g
- Saturated Fat: ~3g
- Sugars: ~8g
- Cholesterol: ~185mg (if egg is included

Jonathan Waxman's Kale Salad

SERVES 4

Ingredients

- 1 pound fresh kale, baby if possible, or the youngest dinosaur kale available
- 4 leaves basil
- 2 cloves garlic, smashed

- 2 salt-cured anchovies, rinsed and filleted
- 1 egg yolk
- 1 tablespoon Dijon mustard
- 1 tablespoon lemon juice (about ¼ of a large lemon)
- ¼ cup extra-virgin olive oil
- Iodized sea salt and pepper, to taste
- 1 ounce grated Pecorino-Romano cheese
- 1 tablespoon finely chopped toasted hazelnuts

Directions
- Wash the kale thoroughly and dry with a salad spinner. On a wooden cutting board, cut the kale into thin ribbons. Transfer the kale to a salad bowl.
- Finely chop the anchovies, garlic, and basil on a cutting board.
- In a separate bowl, combine the basil and garlic combination, the egg, mustard, and lemon juice. Use a whisk to thoroughly combine. Drizzle in the olive oil and whisk vigorously until combined.
- Pour enough dressing over the greens to thoroughly coat it.
- With as much force as possible, crush the kale and dressing with a wooden spoon. (At Barbuto, they use their hands, but they wear gloves!) Season with a pinch of sea salt and black pepper.
- Sprinkle with cheese and nuts.
- Toss thoroughly, taste for flavor, and serve.

Nutritional Information Per Serving
- Calories: ~200-250
- Protein: ~6-8g
- Carbs: ~8-10g
- Fiber: ~4g
- Fat: ~18-22g
- Saturated Fat: ~3-4g
- Sugars: ~2-3g
- Cholesterol: ~110mg

Crab Cakes

SERVES 2

Ingredients

FOR DIPPING SAUCE
- ½ cup avocado mayonnaise, such as Primal Kitchen
- 1 tablespoon capers
- 1 teaspoon diced onion
- 1 tablespoon diced green olives
- Zest of 1 lemon

FOR CRAB CAKES
- 14 ounces of lump crab meat or 14 ounces of hearts of palm (frozen, jarred, or canned and packed in brine, not sugar) drained and finely chopped
- 2 celery stalks, diced
- ½ yellow onion, diced
- 2 cloves garlic, crushed
- 1 teaspoon Old Bay seasoning
- 2 tablespoons cassava flour

- 1 omega-3 or pastured egg or Vegan Egg
- ¼ cup blanched almond flour (Bob's Red Mill makes a great one, available at most grocery stores)
- 3 tablespoons avocado oil

Directions

- First, prepare the sauce by combining all of the ingredients in a small bowl. Cover and chill until needed.
- In a large mixing bowl, combine the crab, celery, onion, garlic, Old Bay seasoning, cassava flour, and egg. The mixture should readily form cakes in your palms. If it's crumbling, add more cassava, 1 teaspoon at a time, until it holds together.
- Divide the crab mixture into four evenly sized cakes. Gently dust the outside of each cake with almond flour, then place it in the refrigerator for 15 to 20 minutes, or until it holds together.
- In a large skillet, heat the avocado oil over medium high heat. Cook the crab cakes for 3 to 4 minutes, or until they are golden. Cook for 3 to 4 minutes more, flipping gently.
- Reduce the heat to low and continue cooking until a sharp knife inserted into the center of one of the cakes comes out heated (1 to 2 minutes).
- Serve with sauce.

Nutritional Information Per Serving
- Calories: ~350-400
- Protein: ~20-25g
- Carbs: ~10-15g
- Fiber: ~3-4g
- Fat: ~30-35g
- Saturated Fat: ~3-4g
- Cholesterol: ~160mg

Halibut with Mushroom Ragout and Lentils

SERVES 4

Ingredients

FOR THE LENTILS
- 2 tablespoons avocado oil
- ½ cup shallots, peeled and finely diced
- 2 cloves of garlic, peeled and sliced paper-thin
- 1 cup lentils
- 2½ cups mushroom stock or Vegetable Stock
- 2 tablespoons dried porcini mushroom powder, finely ground (make your own by pulsing dried porcinis in a spice grinder)*
- 2 tablespoons agave syrup
- Iodized sea salt, to taste
- Freshly ground black pepper, to taste

FOR THE RAGOUT
- 2 tablespoons avocado oil
- ½ pound chanterelle mushrooms, stems trimmed and caps torn into large pieces; cut 2 tablespoons of the firmest mushrooms into fine strips and reserve for the salad
- Small bunch of scallions, green tops cut on angle for garnish, white bottoms sliced thin for sauté
- ½ cup dry white wine
- Drizzle of balsamic vinegar
- 2 tablespoons Parmigiano-Reggiano, finely grated

FOR THE FISH
- 2 tablespoons of ground coriander seed
- Iodized sea salt, to taste
- Freshly ground black pepper, to taste
- 4 halibut center filets (thicker), 4 to 5 ounces each
- ½ cup cilantro

Directions
- Preheat the oven to 425° Fahrenheit.
- Cook the lentils in a large skillet over medium heat, adding the avocado oil and shallots. Cook, stirring periodically, until transparent.
- Bring the garlic, lentils, stock, porcini powder, and agave syrup to a quick boil. Season liberally with sea salt and pepper. Transfer the ingredients to your pressure cooker and secure the top. Pressure cook on high for 15 minutes. Take off the heat and give the pressure cooker ten minutes or so to naturally release the pressure.
- Make the ragout by heating 2 tablespoons of avocado oil in a large skillet over high heat. Cook the huge chanterelles and scallion whites until browned, which should take around 5 minutes. Cook for about 2 minutes after adding the balsamic vinegar and white wine. Stir to mix in the scallion greens and the cooked lentils. Season with sea salt and freshly ground pepper. Add the Parmigiano cheese and stir.
- Prepare the fish. Coriander, sea salt, and pepper should be used to season the halibut's surfaces. Heat a few drops of avocado oil in a medium-sized skillet over high heat. Sear the halibut for about 2 minutes before turning the filets over. Cook the filets on the lower rack of the oven for approximately 6 minutes, depending on thickness and desired doneness.
- To serve, place the halibut on top of the lentil ragout with mushrooms that has been spooned into the middle of the plate. In a small bowl, stir together the cilantro and raw chanterelle julienne, seasoning with sea salt and pepper. Serve on top of the halibut. Serve and enjoy.

Nutritional Information Per Serving

- Calories: ~400-450
- Protein: ~40-45g
- Carbs: ~30-35g
- Fiber: ~10-12g
- Fat: ~15-20g
- Saturated Fat: ~2-3g
- Cholesterol: ~60-70mg

Thai Lemongrass "Meat" Balls

SERVES 4

Ingredients
- 1 tablespoon sesame oil
- 1 tablespoon fresh ginger, minced
- 1 clove garlic, minced
- 1 stalk lemongrass, dry layers removed, thinly sliced
- 1 teaspoon Thai red curry paste
- 1 bag Quorn grounds, thawed, or 12 ounces grass-fed ground beef
- 1 small sweet potato, baked, skin removed, and mashed (about ½ cup)
- 1 omega-3 or pastured egg or Vegan Egg
- 2 tablespoon cassava flour
- 2 tablespoons avocado oil
- 1 can coconut milk
- 1 tablespoon coconut aminos
- Steamed cauliflower rice, for serving

Directions
- Preheat a small skillet over medium-high heat. Saute the sesame oil, ginger, garlic, and lemongrass for about 2 minutes, stirring regularly, until very aromatic.
- Cook for one minute more after adding the curry paste.
- Transfer the mixture to a food processor work bowl, then add the Quorn and sweet potato and pulse until well incorporated (the mixture should be slightly chunky).
- Transfer to a mixing basin, then add the egg and cassava flour. The mixture should be able to be shaped into balls. If the mixture is too loose, gradually add additional flour, one teaspoon at a time, until it is more cohesive.
- Scoop the mixture into tablespoon-sized balls with your fingertips or an ice cream scoop. Refrigerate for 20 minutes.
- Heat the avocado oil in a large skillet over medium-high heat. After the balls have chilled, put them to the pan and cook, stirring periodically, until browned on all sides, about 5 to 7 minutes.
- Cook for 5 minutes, adding the coconut milk and coconut aminos, until the sauce thickens slightly.
- Serve with cooked cauliflower rice.

Nutritional Information Per Serving
- Calories: ~300-350
- Protein: ~15-20g
- Carbs: ~25-30g
- Fiber: ~4-6g
- Fat: ~20-25g

- Saturated Fat: ~7-8g
- Cholesterol: ~60-70mg

Moroccan-Spiced Chicken with Millet Tabbouleh

SERVES 4

Ingredients

FOR THE CHICKEN
- 2 cups coconut yogurt, plain
- Juice of 1 lemon
- Zest of 1 lemon
- Zest of 1 orange
- ½ teaspoon cinnamon
- ½ teaspoon cumin
- ½ teaspoon paprika
- ½ teaspoon black pepper
- ½ teaspoon turmeric
- ½ teaspoon iodized sea salt
- 4 pasture-raised chicken thighs

FOR THE TABBOULEH
- 2 cups cooked millet
- ½ cup minced parsley
- ½ cup minced mint
- ¼ cup minced dill
- 1 teaspoon iodized sea salt
- 1 tablespoon extra-virgin olive oil
- Juice of 1 lemon
- ¼ cup red wine vinegar

Directions

- Marinate the chicken: Mix together the yogurt, lemon juice, lemon zest, orange zest, and spices in a big ziplock bag. Marinate the chicken for at least an hour. (If you're using tempeh, marinate it in the same way for 30 minutes).
- Preheat the oven to 375° Fahrenheit. Spray oil onto a broiler pan or sheet tray with a wire rack. Set aside.
- Make the tabbouleh by combining all of the ingredients in a large bowl and stirring thoroughly. Allow the flavors to mingle for at least 20 minutes (ideal timing for cooking the chicken).
- Take out the marinated chicken (or tempeh), pat dry with paper towels, and place on the baking sheet that has been prepared. If your chicken has skin, put it skin-side down.
- The chicken should be baked for 20 to 25 minutes, then turned over and baked for another 10 to 15 minutes, skin side up, until the meat is 160°F and the skin is crisp. Remove from heat and allow it rest for 5 minutes before serving.
- If using tempeh, bake it for 12 to 15 minutes, turning it over once or twice, until it's crispy. Serve right away after removing from the heat.

Nutritional Information Per Serving
- Calories: ~350-400
- Protein: ~30-35g
- Carbs: ~25-30g

- Fiber: ~4-6g
- Fat: ~18-20g
- Saturated Fat: ~5-7g
- Cholesterol: ~90-100mg

Cauliflower Rice Risotto

SERVES 8

Ingredients

- ¼ cup avocado oil
- 6 cups assorted mushrooms
- 2 medium leeks, rinsed and finely sliced
- ¼ cup minced shallots
- 1 16-ounce package cauliflower rice
- 3 tablespoons arrowroot starch
- 16 ounces mushroom broth or Bone Broth
- 1 can coconut cream
- Juice of 1 lemon
- Zest of 1 lemon
- ¼ cup nutritional yeast or grated Parmigiano-Reggiano cheese
- Salt and pepper, to taste

Directions

- Preheat a dry pan on high. Add oil to the heated pan.
- Sauté the mushrooms until golden brown (10 minutes, stirring infrequently—allow them to brown!)
- Cook the leeks, shallots, and a pinch of salt until transparent, about 4 to 5 minutes.
- Sauté the cauliflower rice for 5 minutes, then whisk in the arrowroot for 1 minute.
- Bring the risotto to a boil, then stir in the mushroom broth or bone broth; it should thicken quickly (2 to 3 minutes).
- Once the mixture has boiled and thickened, add the coconut cream and reduce the heat to just simmer.
- Season with lemon juice, lemon zest, nutritional yeast, or grated Parmigiano-Reggiano, to taste. Serve warm.

Nutritional Information Per Serving
- Calories: ~200-250
- Protein: ~4-5g
- Carbs: ~14-18g
- Fiber: ~5-6g
- Fat: ~18-22g
- Saturated Fat: ~10-12g
- Cholesterol: ~5-10mg

Cauliflower-Ginger Fried Rice

SERVES 6 TO 8

Ingredients

- 2½ tablespoons sesame oil
- 1 medium yellow onion, diced
- 1 1-inch piece ginger root, peeled and minced
- 2 cloves garlic, minced
- 8 to 12 dried shiitake mushrooms, reconstituted in hot water and cut

- into thin strips
- 4 ounces water chestnuts, roughly chopped
- 4 celery stalks, thinly sliced
- 32 ounces cauliflower rice (approximately 4 cups)
- 1 tablespoon coconut aminos
- ¼ teaspoon powdered mustard
- ¼ teaspoon cayenne pepper (optional)
- 2 omega-3 or pastured eggs or Vegan Eggs, whisked (optional)

Directions
- In a large skillet or wok, warm the sesame oil over medium-high heat.
- Cook the onion and ginger for 3 to 4 minutes, or until the onions are transparent. Cook for an additional 2 to 3 minutes, until the garlic is aromatic.
- After adding the celery and water chestnuts, simmer for 3 to 4 minutes, or until the vegetables are tender.
- Increase the heat to high and mix in the cauliflower rice. Cook for another 3 to 4 minutes, stirring regularly to keep it from burning.
- Add 1 tablespoon coconut aminos, followed by the mustard powder and cayenne, if using.
- Cook over high heat, tossing regularly, until the cauliflower is soft but not mushy.
- If using eggs, create a well in the cauliflower rice and fill with the whisked eggs. Once they've started to cook, mix them into the cauliflower rice. Once the eggs have set, remove from the pan and serve.

Nutritional Information Per Serving
- Calories: ~120-150
- Protein: ~5-6g
- Carbs: ~10-12g
- Fiber: ~4-5g
- Fat: ~9-11g
- Saturated Fat: ~1-2g
- Cholesterol: ~70-80mg

Sweet Potato Spaghetti and Meatballs

SERVES 4

Ingredients
- 1 tablespoon salt
- 1 pound ground kosher turkey
- ½ brown onion, minced
- 1 clove garlic, crushed
- 1 omega-3 or pastured egg or Vegan Egg
- 1 tablespoon Worcestershire sauce or coconut aminos
- ⅓ cup cassava flour
- 1 large sweet potato (about 1 pound), peeled and spiralized
- 1 tablespoon extra-virgin olive oil
- 4 cups baby spinach
- 1 cup vegetable broth
- 1 cup Classic Basil Pesto

Directions

- Bring a big saucepan of water to a boil with a tablespoon of salt.
- Combine turkey, onion, garlic, egg or VeganEgg, Worcestershire sauce, coconut aminos, and cassava flour. For the meatballs to come together, the mixture must be sufficiently thick. If not, add more cassava flour, half a teaspoon at a time.
- Form the beef mixture into little balls, each containing roughly two teaspoons. Place in the refrigerator for 15 minutes.
- When the water reaches a boil, add the sweet potato noodles. Cook until soft, about 5 minutes; then, take out of water and set aside.
- Cook in a large skillet over medium heat. Cook the meatballs, rotating regularly, until they are golden brown on all sides.
- Cover the pan and reduce the heat to low. Add the spinach and vegetable broth. Continue cooking for ten more minutes, or until the spinach has wilted and the meatballs are thoroughly cooked.
- Combine the "noodles" and toss. Remove from the heat and carefully fold in the pesto before serving.

Nutritional Information Per Serving

- Calories: ~350-400
- Protein: ~30-35g
- Carbs: ~25-30g
- Fiber: ~6-8g
- Fat: ~20-25g
- Saturated Fat: ~3-4g
- Cholesterol: ~100-120mg

Greens with Eggs and Ham

SERVES 1

Ingredients

- ¼ cup Classic Balsamic Vinaigrette
- 2 cups mixed baby greens
- ½ cup thinly sliced fennel
- 1 cup broccoli slaw
- 1 cup diced artichoke hearts (frozen and thawed)
- ½ avocado, cubed
- 1 tablespoon extra-virgin olive oil
- 2 omega-3 or pastured eggs or the other half of the avocado
- 2 ounces prosciutto, diced (optional)

Directions

- Mix the vinaigrette, greens, fennel, slaw, and artichoke hearts in a large bowl until well blended.
- Toss in the avocado cubes until evenly coated. Set aside.
- In a small skillet, warm the olive oil over medium heat. Cook the eggs until they are overeasy, then remove from heat.
- Place the greens in a serving bowl, then add the egg and prosciutto, if using.

Nutritional Information Per Serving
- Calories: ~400-450
- Protein: ~20-25g
- Carbs: ~15-18g
- Fiber: ~8-10g
- Fat: ~30-35g
- Saturated Fat: ~5-6g
- Cholesterol: ~220-250mg

Chapter 8

Vegetables and Sides

Crispy Brussels Sprouts with Balsamic and Dates

SERVES 4

Ingredients
- 1 pound Brussels sprouts, stems removed, cut in half
- ½ cup avocado oil or olive oil
- 2 teaspoons iodized sea salt, divided
- 1 tablespoon balsamic reduction*
- ½ cup pitted dates, finely chopped
- Juice of ½ lemon
- ½ cup slivered toasted almond

Directions
- Preheat the oven to 350° Fahrenheit.
- Line a baking sheet with a single layer of Brussels sprouts that have been halved and tossed in oil. Sprinkle with salt.
- Bake for 20 to 30 minutes, or until the Brussels sprouts are golden and slightly crunchy on the outside yet soft on the inside.
- Allow the sprouts to cool down. While still heated, combine the balsamic reduction, salt, sliced dates, lemon juice, and toasted almonds.
- Mix thoroughly, and serve warm.

Nutritional Information Per Serving
- Calories: ~220-250
- Protein: ~5g
- Carbs: ~30g
- Fiber: ~7g
- Fat: ~14g
- Saturated Fat: ~2g
- Cholesterol: ~0mg

Dr. G's Lectin-Light Caprese Salad

SERVES 4

Ingredients
- 3 large tomatoes
- 2 cups salad greens (for serving)
- ¼ cup extra-virgin olive oil
- 2 tablespoons Classic Basil Pesto
- 1 cup basil leaves
- 8 ounces buffalo mozzarella

- ¼ cup balsamic vinegar
- ½ teaspoon iodized sea salt

Directions
- First, prepare the tomatoes by peeling them with a serrated vegetable peeler and then cutting them in half. Using a spoon, carefully scrape off the seeds and pulp from the tomatoes, then slice them with a serrated knife.
- Toss the leaves in a big salad basin with the olive oil and pesto.
- Put the tomatoes, basil leaves, and mozzarella on top of the greens.
- Serve with a drizzle of balsamic vinegar and sea salt.

Nutritional Information Per Serving
- Calories: ~250-280
- Protein: ~12g
- Carbs: ~10g
- Fiber: ~2g
- Fat: ~20g
- Saturated Fat: ~6g
- Cholesterol: ~30mg

Herb-Roasted Radishes

SERVES 4

Ingredients
- 1½ pound radishes, stems trimmed, quartered
- 4 tablespoons French or Italian grass fed butter (such as Trader Joe's Cultured French Butter, President, or Beurre D'Insigny), melted, or avocado oil
- 1 teaspoon iodized sea salt
- ¼ cup minced parsley
- ¼ cup minced mint

Directions
- Preheat the oven to 425° Fahrenheit.
- Mix the radishes with half the butter or oil.
- Spread out in a single layer on a sheet tray and season with salt.
- Bake for 20–25 minutes, or until tender.
- While the radishes are roasting, warm the remaining butter or oil in a small skillet over medium-high heat. When heated, stir in the herbs and remove from the heat.
- Straight onto the sheet tray, remove the radishes from the oven skillet and combine with the herb mixture. Serve either hot or room temperature.

Nutritional Information Per Serving
- Calories: ~150-170
- Protein: ~2g
- Carbs: ~10g
- Fiber: ~4g
- Fat: ~12g
- Saturated Fat: ~4g
- Cholesterol: ~20mg

Thanksgiving Millet Stuffing

SERVES 4 TO 6

Ingredients

- ¼ cup plus 1 tablespoon French or Italian grass-fed butter (such as Trader Joe's Cultured French Butter, President, or Beurre D'Insigny) or olive oil spray for pan
- 3 cups cooked millet (prepared according to package instructions)
- 2 yellow onions, finely diced
- 3 carrots, finely diced
- 3 celery stalks, finely diced
- 5 cloves garlic, minced
- 1½ tablespoons minced fresh sage
- 1 tablespoon minced fresh parsley
- 2 tablespoons dried poultry seasoning (no salt added)
- 1 pound mushrooms, finely diced
- 1 teaspoon minced fresh thyme
- ½ teaspoon sea salt
- ½ teaspoon ground black pepper

Directions

- Preheat the oven to 350° Fahrenheit. Prepare a 9 x 13-inch casserole dish by buttering it or spraying it with 1 tablespoon of olive oil.
- Place the cooked millet in a large mixing basin, and put aside.
- In a large skillet or wok, melt half of the butter or oil over medium-high heat. Cook the carrots, celery, and onions until soft, stirring frequently.
- Cook for 2 to 3 minutes more, stirring in the garlic, sage, parsley, and poultry seasoning until aromatic. Add to the basin containing the millet.
- In the same skillet, heat the remaining oil or butter and add mushrooms and thyme. Cook the mushrooms till golden brown and soft, then stir them into the millet mixture.
- Stir in the stuffing mixture until combined. Season the dish with salt and pepper.
- Bake the stuffing in the baking dish for 25 to 35 minutes, or until the top is golden brown and the filling is heated throughout.

Nutritional Information Per Serving (Approximate)
- Calories: ~220-250
- Protein: ~6g
- Carbs: ~30g
- Fiber: ~4g
- Fat: ~8g
- Saturated Fat: ~3g
- Cholesterol: ~10mg (if using butter)
- Sodium: ~250mg

Wild Rice Salad

SERVES 4

Ingredients

- ¼ cup plus 1 tablespoon extra-virgin olive oil

- 1 onion, diced
- 2 cups wild rice
- 3 cups Vegetable Stock
- ½ cup roasted pine nuts
- 6 green onions or scallions, chopped
- 8 ounces crumbled goat feta (optional)
- Iodized sea salt and pepper, to taste

Directions
- Put 1 tablespoon of olive oil in a pressure cooker and set it over medium-high heat on the stove (or on the electric pressure cooker's sauté setting).
- Cook the onion until soft, then add the rice and sauté for another 2 to 3 minutes.
- Put the rice in the pressure cooker and add the broth. Cook for thirty minutes.
- When done, leave the cover on for 1 to 2 hours to allow the rice to cook on its own heat.
- Pour the remaining quarter cup of olive oil over the rice, followed by the pine nuts, green onion or scallions, and feta, if using. Stir to mix.
- Adjust the seasoning with salt and pepper. Serve either warm or at room temperature.

Nutritional Information Per Serving (Approximate)
- Calories: ~400
- Protein: ~10g (varies depending on feta inclusion)
- Carbs: ~35g
- Fiber: ~5g
- Fat: ~25g
- Saturated Fat: ~5g (higher with feta)
- Sodium: ~300mg (varies with broth and feta)

Spiced Carrot and Broccoli Slaw

SERVES 4 TO 6

Ingredients
- 2 cups broccoli slaw
- 1 cup shredded red cabbage
- 2 cups shredded carrots
- 1 cup pickled red onions
- ¼ cup extra-virgin olive oil
- 2 cloves garlic, minced
- 1 tablespoon minced ginger
- ½ teaspoon cinnamon
- 1 teaspoon paprika
- ½ teaspoon cumin
- 1 teaspoon turmeric
- 1 teaspoon iodized sea salt
- 2 cups coconut or goat's milk yogurt

Directions
- To a large mixing bowl, combine the broccoli slaw, red cabbage, carrots, and pickled red onions.
- Heat the ginger, garlic, and olive oil in a small sauté pan over medium heat until fragrant. Cook for a further 30 seconds to 1 minute, until

- the cinnamon, paprika, cumin, turmeric, and sea salt have roasted.
- Whisk in the yogurt after removing it from the heat. Combine the yogurt and slaw, and serve at room temperature (or cooled).

Nutritional Information (per serving, approximate for 6 servings):
- Calories: 120
- Protein: 3g
- Carbohydrates: 10g
- Fiber: 3g
- Sugar: 5g
- Fat: 8g
- Saturated Fat: 3g
- Sodium: 370mg
- Calcium: 60mg
- Iron: 1mg

Prosciutto-Braised Cabbage

SERVES 4

Ingredients
- 2 tablespoons extra-virgin olive oil
- 1 1½-pound head of green cabbage, cut through the core into 6 wedges
- ½ cup chopped prosciutto, preferably Prosciutto di Parma (optional)
- 1 medium onion, thinly sliced
- ½ cup apple cider vinegar
- 1 cup Vegetable Stock
- 1 teaspoon iodized sea salt
- ¼ cup pomegranate molasses

Directions
- In a big, deep skillet, heat the olive oil until it shimmers.
- Cook the cabbage wedges, cut side down, over medium heat for 6 to 8 minutes, stirring periodically to avoid scorching. Set aside.
- Cook the prosciutto and onion in the skillet over medium heat, stirring periodically, until the onions are soft and the prosciutto begins to crisp.
- Stir in the vinegar and cook over medium-high heat for about 3 minutes, or until reduced by half. Bring the stock and salt to a boil.
- Put the cabbage wedges back in the skillet, cover, and cook over medium-low heat for about 20 minutes, rotating once, until they are soft.
- Transfer the cabbage to a plate with a slotted spoon or spatula and cover with foil until ready to serve.
- Drizzle with pomegranate molasses before serving.

Nutritional Information (per serving, approximate for 4 servings):
- Calories: 130
- Protein: 3g
- Carbohydrates: 16g
- Fiber: 4g
- Sugar: 9g
- Fat: 7g
- Saturated Fat: 1g

- Sodium: 470mg
- Calcium: 50mg
- Iron: 1mg

Ralph's Roasted Cauliflower

SERVES 4 TO 5

Ingredients
- ¼ cup plus 3 tablespoons extra-virgin olive oil
- 1 head cauliflower, green leaves discarded
- 1 teaspoon iodized sea salt
- 1 tablespoon fresh lemon juice, or to taste
- 1 tablespoon drained small capers
- 1 teaspoon monk-fruit sweetener or 1 packet stevia
- ¼ teaspoon black pepper
- ¼ cup chopped fresh flat-leaf parsley (optional)

Directions
- The oven should be preheated to 450°F. Place an oven rack in the middle. Lightly grease a 9-inch pie plate or square baking dish.
- Remove only the core of the cauliflower, keeping the head intact, and arrange it in a pie plate or baking dish, core side down.
- Sprinkle half a teaspoon of salt and 3 tablespoons of olive oil over the cauliflower before putting the baking dish or pie plate in the oven.
- Bake until soft, 1 hour to 1 hour and 15 minutes (duration varies depending on oven and cauliflower size; check tenderness frequently). Cauliflower should appear somewhat browned. Once finished, transfer to a serving plate.
- In a separate bowl, combine the lemon juice, capers, monk-fruit sweetener or stevia, pepper, and the remaining half teaspoon salt. Whisk in the remaining quarter cup oil.
- Sprinkle the cauliflower with the parsley, if using, and drizzle with drissing.

Nutritional Information (per serving, approximate for 5 servings):
- Calories: 150
- Protein: 2g
- Carbohydrates: 9g
- Fiber: 3g
- Sugar: 3g
- Fat: 14g
- Saturated Fat: 2g
- Sodium: 430mg
- Calcium: 30mg
- Iron: 0.5mg

Spicy Sweet Potato Fritters

SERVES 8 TO 10

Ingredients

- 5 cups peeled and spiralized sweet potatoes
- ¼ cup tapioca flour
- ¼ cup almond flour
- ½ cup thinly sliced scallions
- ½ cup minced shallots
- ½ teaspoon cayenne pepper
- 1 or 2 pinches of cumin
- 2 omega-3 or pastured eggs or Vegan Eggs
- 1 to 2 cups coconut oil (for cooking)
- 1 teaspoon iodized sea salt

Directions

- Place the sweet potatoes in a large basin and cut them into 1- or 2-inch pieces using kitchen scissors.
- Combine the tapioca flour, almond flour, scallions, shallots, cayenne pepper, cumin, and eggs.
- Mix until the potatoes are evenly covered in flour and the mixture holds together properly.
- Form into little patties about 4 inches in diameter.
- In a large skillet, melt 2 to 3 tablespoons coconut oil over medium heat.
- When the oil is hot, put the patties on the skillet. The patties should be cooked for 4 to 6 minutes, or until golden brown, then turned over and cooked for 2 more minutes on each side. (For each consecutive batch, increase the amount of coconut oil in the skillet.)
- These are best served straight off the griddle, sprinkled with sea salt.

Nutritional Information (per serving, approximate for 10 servings):

- Calories: 160
- Protein: 2g
- Carbohydrates: 14g
- Fiber: 2g
- Sugar: 3g
- Fat: 11g
- Saturated Fat: 7g
- Sodium: 240mg
- Calcium: 20mg
- Iron: 0.6mg

Sweet and Sour Cabbage and Kale Slaw

SERVES 4

Ingredients

- 2 cups thinly sliced kale, ribs removed
- ½ teaspoon iodized sea salt
- 1 cup coconut yogurt
- 1 tablespoon Dijon mustard
- Juice of 1 lemon
- 1 teaspoon garlic powder
- ½ teaspoon paprika
- 2 tablespoons pomegranate molasses or balsamic reduction
- 2 cups thinly sliced cabbage
- 1 red onion, thinly sliced

½ cup dried figs (no sugar added), diced

Directions
- In a large dish, toss the kale with salt until soft.
- In a small mixing bowl, combine the yogurt, Dijon mustard, lemon juice, garlic powder, paprika, and pomegranate molasses/balsamic reduction.
- Toss the kale with the dressing, cabbage, onion, and figs to incorporate.
- Serve either cold or at room temperature.

Nutritional Information (per serving, approximate):
- Calories: 110
- Protein: 3g
- Carbohydrates: 16g
- Fiber: 4g
- Sugar: 9g
- Fat: 4g
- Saturated Fat: 3g
- Sodium: 250mg
- Calcium: 60mg
- Iron: 1mg

Chapter 9

Sweet Bites

Almond Delight Grasshopper Ice Cream

MAKES 1 QUART

Ingredients
- 2 15-ounce cans unsweetened coconut cream
- ½ cup Swerve sweetener or 10 pitted dates
- ½ teaspoon vanilla extract
- 1 ripe avocado
- ½ cup unsweetened coconut flakes
- ½ cup slivered toasted almonds
- ½ cup chopped bittersweet chocolate (at least 72 percent cacao)

Directions
- Check that the bowl of your ice cream machine is thoroughly frozen.
- In a large saucepan, combine the coconut cream, Swerve sweetener or dates, and vanilla essence. Simmer on medium until the mixture is warmed through and the sweetener, if used, has dissolved.
- Combine the avocado and coconut cream in a high-speed blender or food processor fitted with an S-blade until smooth.
- Refrigerate the mixture for at least 4 hours, preferably overnight.
- Follow the freezing directions on your ice cream machine. When the ice cream is nearly frozen, stir in the coconut flakes, toasted almonds, and chocolate.
- Eat with a soft-serve consistency or freeze in an airtight container for 1 to 2 hours before serving.
- **Note:** After a few hours in the freezer, this ice cream becomes quite hard, so let it defrost until scoopable.

Nutritional Information (per serving, approximate):
- Calories: 280
- Protein: 4g
- Carbohydrates: 12g
- Fiber: 5g
- Sugar: 5g
- Fat: 26g
- Saturated Fat: 20g

Pistachio Ice Cream

MAKES 1 GENEROUS PINT

Ingredients

- 2 cups coconut cream
- ½ cup Swerve (erythritol)
- 1 vanilla bean, split
- 1 cup roasted shelled pistachios (unsalted, if possible)
- 1 large avocado, skin and pit removed
- ¼ teaspoon iodized sea salt (unless using salted pistachios)

Directions

- Heat the coconut cream, Swerve, and vanilla bean over low heat (if possible, keep it simmering) for around 5 to 10 minutes until Swerve melts.
- To infuse flavor, add the pistachios and cook on low heat for 20 to 30 minutes.
- Transfer the contents to a high-speed blender and puree until smooth.
- Blend in the avocado and sea salt until the mixture is smooth.
- Chill in the refrigerator until extremely cold, then freeze according to the manufacturer's directions for your ice cream maker.
- Serve immediately with a soft-serve consistency or place in the freezer to set further.
- **Note:** Because this freezes firmly, it to thaw at room temperature before scooping.

Nutritional Information (per serving, approximate):
- Calories: 260
- Protein: 4g
- Carbohydrates: 10g
- Fiber: 4g
- Sugar: 2g
- Fat: 23g
- Saturated Fat: 16g
- Sodium: 90mg
- Calcium: 25mg
- Iron: 1.5mg

Lemon Poppy Coffee Cake

SERVES 8

Ingredients

- olive oil spray
- 1½ cups almond flour
- ¼ cup coconut flour
- ½ teaspoon salt
- 1 teaspoon baking soda
- 3 omega-3 or pastured eggs or VeganEggs
- ½ cup Swerve (erythritol)
- ¼ cup avocado oil
- Juice of 3 lemons
- Zest of 2 lemons
- ¼ cup unsweetened coconut milk
- 1 teaspoon vanilla extract
- 2 tablespoons poppy seeds

Directions

- Line a 9 x 5-inch loaf pan with parchment paper after spraying it with olive oil. Preheat the oven to 350° Fahrenheit.
- In a mixing dish, combine almond flour, coconut flour, salt, and baking soda.
- In a separate bowl, mix together the eggs, Swerve, avocado oil, lemon juice, lemon zest, coconut milk, and vanilla essence.
- Whisk together the wet and dry ingredients until completely blended.
- Fold in the poppy seeds, and then transfer the dough to the prepared loaf pan.
- Bake for 35–40 minutes, or until a toothpick inserted into the center of the loaf comes out clean.
- Allow it cool for a few minutes before removing the loaf by running a knife around the pan's edge. Serve when still heated or at room temperature.

Nutritional Information (per serving, approximate):

- Calories: 220
- Protein: 6g
- Carbohydrates: 9g
- Fiber: 3g
- Sugar: 1g
- Fat: 19g
- Saturated Fat: 3g
- Sodium: 190mg
- Calcium: 40mg

Chocolate Cream Pie

SERVES 8

Ingredients

- 1 Plant Paradox Piecrust, baked
- ½ cup coconut cream
- ⅔ cup granulated Swerve (erythritol)
- 2 ounces bittersweet chocolate (72 percent cacao or higher)
- 3 large ripe avocados, peeled and pitted
- ½ cup high-quality unsweetened cocoa powder
- 2 teaspoons pure vanilla extract
- ¼ teaspoon salt
- Fresh, in-season fruit for serving (I suggest figs or berries

Directions

- In a small saucepan, combine the coconut cream, Swerve, and chocolate, stirring constantly until the chocolate melts and the Swerve dissolves. Set aside.
- Blend the avocado, coconut cream mixture, cocoa powder, vanilla extract, and salt in a high-speed blender or food processor equipped with an S-blade until smooth.
- Transfer to the prepared pie shell, smoothing the filling evenly on top.
- Wrap tightly and chill for at least 2 hours, or up to 2 days, before serving.
- Allow it to come to room temperature before slicing, or use a

- hot knife to easily cut through the chocolate and serve with fresh fruit. Leftovers should be refrigerated, but let the pie come to room temperature before serving.

Nutritional Information (per serving, approximate):
- Calories: 220
- Protein: 3g
- Carbohydrates: 15g
- Fiber: 6g
- Sugar: 2g
- Fat: 18g
- Saturated Fat: 8g
- Sodium: 120mg

Chocolate Mint Cookies

MAKES 12 LARGE OR 18 SMALL COOKIES

Ingredients
- 1 cup creamy almond butter
- ⅔ cup confectioner's Swerve (erythritol)
- 2 tablespoons non-Dutched cocoa powder
- 2 tablespoons blanched almond meal
- 1 tablespoon coconut flour
- 2 tablespoons water
- 2 large omega-3 or pastured eggs or VeganEggs
- 2 tablespoons melted, salted butter or coconut oil
- 1½ teaspoons pure peppermint extract
- 1 teaspoon baking soda
- ¼ cup chopped bittersweet chocolate

Directions
- Preheat the oven to 350° Fahrenheit. Using parchment paper or a silicone baking mat (a Silpat), line a rimmed baking sheet.
- In a large mixing bowl, whisk together almond butter, erythritol, cocoa powder, almond meal, coconut flour, water, eggs, butter or oil, peppermint essence, and baking soda.
- Mix all ingredients together with a stand mixer fitted with the paddle attachment or a whisk and some considerable arm power.
- Fold in the chocolate pieces.
- To make twelve cookies, roll out the cookie dough into 2-inch balls; to make eighteen, roll it out slightly smaller.
- With space to spread, place the cookie-dough balls on the baking sheet that has been prepared.
- Bake for 10–12 minutes. Allow the cookies to cool before eating. Keep any leftovers in an airtight container for 3-4 days.

Nutritional Information (per cookie, approximate for 12 cookies):
- Calories: 140
- Protein: 4g

- Carbohydrates: 7g
- Fiber: 3g
- Sugar: 1g
- Fat: 12g
- Saturated Fat: 3g
- Sodium: 95mg

Dried Fig "Truffles"

MAKES 12

Ingredients

- 12 whole dried unsweetened figs
- 1 cup boiling water
- 1 cup coconut cream
- Zest of 1 orange
- 1 tablespoon chopped rosemary
- 1 cup chopped bittersweet chocolate, at least 72 percent cacao

Directions

- Allow the figs to soak in boiling water until malleable, about 20 minutes.
- Pat the figs dry with a kitchen towel and leave aside.
- In a small saucepan, combine the coconut cream, orange zest, and rosemary. Bring to a simmer.
- Whisk in chocolate until melted after lowering the heat to very low.
- Allow the chocolate mixture to cool to room temperature before transferring to a pastry bag fitted with a round tip.
- Fill the figs with chocolate cream from the bottom (the figs will have a little hole in the bottom that is ideal for stuffing) until they are filled.
- Allow the figs to set before serving; this will take 6 to 8 hours at room temperature or 2 to 4 hours in the fridge. (Before serving, allow them to reach room temperature.)

Nutritional Information (per truffle, approximate for 12 truffles):
- Calories: 140
- Protein: 1g
- Carbohydrates: 22g
- Fiber: 4g
- Sugar: 18g
- Fat: 9g
- Saturated Fat: 6g
- Sodium: 5m

Funnel Cake with Blueberry Sauce

SERVES 4

Ingredients

FOR THE SAUCE
- 2 cups wild blueberries (frozen okay)
- 1 teaspoon coconut oil
- Zest of 1 lemon
- Juice of 1 lemon
- ½ teaspoon cinnamon
- 8 to 10 drops stevia

FOR THE FUNNEL CAKES
- 1 cup tapioca flour

- 2 pastured or omega-3 eggs or VeganEggs
- 2 tablespoon yacón syrup or
- 1 tablespoon Swerve (erythritol)
- 2 tablespoon avocado oil
- Pinch of iodized sea salt
- Avocado oil for frying

Directions
- First, prepare the blueberry sauce by combining all of the ingredients in a small saucepan and cooking over low heat for about 5 minutes, or until the blueberries release their juices.
- In a blender, transfer the blueberry sauce and pulse until it becomes semi-smooth. Set away until needed.
- In a mixing bowl, combine the tapioca flour, eggs, yacón syrup or Swerve, avocado oil, and a pinch of salt. Stir until smooth. Put aside.
- In a small saucepan, pour approximately 1 inch of avocado oil. Heat the oil over medium heat until it shimmers (about 350°F). Transfer the batter to a sandwich bag or pastry bag. Once the oil has shimmered (it is hot enough to fry), snip the tip of the sandwich bag, if using.
- Now, quickly drip the batter into the heated oil, overlapping to create the iconic funnel cake squiggle.
- Allow the underside of the funnel cake to brown for about 1 minute before flipping it over to brown the other side.
- Remove from the oil and set aside on a towel-lined platter.
- Serve hot, drizzling with blueberry sauce.

Total (Funnel Cake + Blueberry Sauce):
- Calories: 280
- Protein: 3.5g
- Carbohydrates: 29g
- Fiber: 3g
- Sugar: 7g
- Fat: 17.5g
- Saturated Fat: 2g
- Sodium: 61mg

Ginger Brownie Bites

SERVES 12 TO 16

Ingredients
- 1 cup over 80 percent cacao chocolate, cut into small pieces
- ¼ cup French or Italian butter, softened, or coconut oil
- ¾ cup monk-fruit sweetener (use a spice grinder to make into powder) or ⅓ cup Swerve (erythritol)
- ½ teaspoon iodized sea salt
- 3 teaspoons grated fresh ginger
- 1 teaspoon almond extract
- 2 large omega-3 or pastured eggs or VeganEggs
- ⅔ cup blanched almond flour
- ⅓ cup tapioca starch

- 1 cup chopped toasted walnuts or toasted slivered almonds (optional)

Directions

- Preheat oven to 325°F and prepare an 8 x 8-inch baking tray with parchment paper.
- Melt the butter or coconut oil and chocolate in a double broiler and stir until smooth.
- Remove from the heat and transfer to a medium mixing bowl with a spatula.
- Mix in the monk fruit powder or Swerve, salt, ginger, and almond essence.
- Let the mixture cool for a few minutes.
- In a second bowl, lightly whisk the eggs before adding the almond flour and tapioca starch.
- Whisk in the chocolate mixture until combined.
- If using, fold roasted walnuts or slivered almonds into the batter.
- Pour the batter into the baking pan you've prepared. Bake for 30 minutes, or until a toothpick comes out clean. Keep leftovers in an airtight jar at room temperature for three to four days.

Nutritional Information (per serving, approximate for 16 servings):
- Calories: 145
- Protein: 3g
- Carbohydrates: 8g
- Fiber: 2g
- Sugar: 1g
- Fat: 12g
- Saturated Fat: 6g
- Sodium: 80mg

Cinnamon Sweet Potato Blondies

MAKES 12

Ingredients
- olive or coconut oil spray
- ⅓ cup coconut oil, softened but not melted
- ⅓ cup yacón syrup or 4 tablespoons confectioner's Swerve (erythritol)
- ½ cup sweet potato puree (from baked sweet potatoes)
- 1 cup coconut milk
- 2 omega-3 or pastured eggs or VeganEggs
- 2 cups blanched almond flour
- 3 tablespoon coconut flour
- ½ teaspoon baking soda
- 1 teaspoon cinnamon
- ¼ teaspoon cloves
- ½ teaspoon vanilla extract
- ½ teaspoon salt

Directions
- Preheat your oven to 350°F. Coat an 8 x 8-inch glass baking dish with olive or coconut oil.
- Cream together the coconut oil and yacón syrup (or Swerve) in a mixing

- bowl or with a stand mixer equipped with a paddle attachment.
- Combine the sweet potato puree, coconut milk, and eggs.
- Combine the flours, baking soda, spices, vanilla extract, and salt; stir thoroughly.
- Evenly distribute the batter in the baking dish that has been prepared.
- Bake for approximately 45 minutes, or until a toothpick inserted into the center comes out clean and the tops are golden brown.
- Allow to cool till room temperature before cutting. For three to four days, store at room temperature in an airtight container.

Nutritional Information (per serving, approximate for 12 servings):
- Calories: 180
- Protein: 4g
- Carbohydrates: 8g
- Fiber: 3g
- Sugar: 2g
- Fat: 15g
- Saturated Fat: 7g
- Sodium: 130mg

Plant Paradox Piecrust

MAKES 2 SINGLE CRUSTS OR 1 DOUBLE CRUST

Ingredients

- 1½ cups plus 1 tablespoon blanched almond flour
- 1½ cups plus 1 tablespoon tapioca starch
- ½ teaspoon monk-fruit sweetener (using spice grinder to make into powder) or 1 packet stevia
- ½ teaspoon baking powder
- ½ teaspoon iodized sea salt
- 1 large omega-3 or pastured egg or VeganEgg
- 5½ tablespoons softened Italian or French butter or coconut oil
- 1 teaspoon champagne vinegar or white balsamic vinegar
- 2 tablespoons cold water, or as needed

Directions
- Almond flour, tapioca starch, monk fruit sweetener (or stevia), baking powder, and salt should all be combined in a food processor. Pulse until well combined, scraping down the sides as needed.
- In a small mixing dish, combine the eggs, butter or coconut oil, and vinegar.
- Pour slowly into a food processor set on low speed.
- Combine and pulse for about 1 minute; the dough will still appear crumbly.
- To ensure the dough maintains its shape, open the food processor and squeeze it with your hands. If the dough is too dry, add cold water one

- teaspoon at a time while continuing to test it.
- Gently knead the dough into a ball after taking it out of the processor.
- If the dough is excessively wet and sticky, add some tapioca starch and knead it.
- Separate the dough into two equal pieces.

TO ROLL OUT AND PAR-BAKE

- Preheat the oven to 350° Fahrenheit. Spray a pie pan generously with olive oil and leave aside.
- Roll out the dough between two sheets of parchment paper into an even circle the size of your pan.
- Remove the top layer of parchment paper and place the pie pan on top. Slide your hand carefully beneath the bottom parchment paper and place your other hand on the pie pan before flipping the dough over and inserting it inside the pie pan.
- Mold the dough into the pie pan while still covered with parchment paper.
- Repair any fractures with your finger, then pierce the inside edge where the pan's wall begins with a fork. Also, pierce the bottom four times (to avoid bubbling).
- Preheat the oven to 350°F, then bake for 30 to 40 minutes, or until gently browned.

Nutritional Information (per serving, approximate for 8 servings per crust):
- Calories: 230
- Protein: 3g
- Carbohydrates: 12g
- Fiber: 2g
- Sugar: 1g
- Fat: 19g
- Saturated Fat: 7g
- Sodium: 120mg

Chapter 10

Sauces, Condiments, and Dressings

Addictive Caramelized Onion Bourbon Jam

MAKES 3 CUPS

Ingredients

- ½ cup sliced nitrate-free pastured bacon (optional)
- ¼ cup extra-virgin olive oil
- 6 large yellow onions, thinly sliced
- ¼ cup fresh thyme leaves
- 1 teaspoon iodized sea salt
- 3 tablespoons bourbon or balsamic vinegar
- 1 tablespoon yacón syrup, or 2 packets stevia

Directions

- If using bacon, cook over medium-low heat until slightly crispy. Place the oil, onions, thyme, and salt in a pan over medium-low heat. Stir frequently to avoid scorching.
- Cook for 20-30 minutes, or until the onions are beautifully golden brown.
- Cook until the bourbon or vinegar, as well as the sugar, have evaporated.
- Transfer the mixture to jars and allow to cool before serving. Jam will last 2 to 3 weeks in the refrigerator.

Nutritional Information (per tablespoon, approximate):
- Calories: 30
- Protein: 0.3g
- Carbohydrates: 3g
- Fiber: 0.5g
- Sugar: 1.5g
- Fat: 2g
- Saturated Fat: 0.3g
- Sodium: 75mg

Classic Basil Pesto

MAKES 1 CUP

Ingredients

- ½ cup toasted pine nuts or blanched toasted almonds
- 3 cloves garlic
- 1 teaspoon iodized sea salt
- ½ cup grated Parmigiano-Reggiano cheese or ¼ cup nutritional yeast

- 3 cups fresh basil leaves, loosely packed
- ¾ cup top quality extra-virgin olive oil

Directions

- Pulse the nuts, garlic, and sea salt in a high-speed blender or food processor equipped with an S-blade until powdered.
- Add the cheese and basil, and pulse until combined, scraping occasionally.
- While the machine is running, drip in the olive oil until well incorporated.
- Use immediately or refrigerate in an airtight container for up to one week.
- If you want to keep your pesto longer, put it in ice cube trays and freeze. After freezing, transfer the cubes to an airtight freezer bag.

Nutritional Information (per tablespoon, approximate):
- Calories: 85
- Protein: 1.5g
- Carbohydrates: 0.5g
- Fiber: 0.2g
- Sugar: 0.1g
- Fat: 9g
- Saturated Fat: 1.5g
- Sodium: 110mg

Plant Paradox Guacamole

SERVES 4 TO 6

Ingredients
- 4 ripe avocados, cut in half, pits removed
- 2 cloves garlic, crushed
- 1 red onion, minced
- ¼ cup cilantro
- 1 teaspoon cumin
- 1 teaspoon iodized sea salt
- Juice of 4 limes
- 1 dash of hot sauce (optional)

Directions
- Place the avocado in a large bowl and mash with a potato masher.
- Stir in the other ingredients until completely combined.
- Taste and adjust the seasoning as necessary.
- Serve with Siete brand grain-free tortilla chips, fresh carrots, sliced jicama, or cassava tortillas (and chips).

Nutritional Information (per serving, based on 6 servings):
- Calories: 220
- Protein: 2.5g
- Carbohydrates: 12g
- Fiber: 8g
- Sugar: 1g
- Fat: 20g
- Saturated Fat: 3g
- Sodium: 400mg

Vegan Caesar Dressing

MAKES 1 CUP

Ingredients
- ½ cup tahini
- 1 garlic clove, crushed
- ¼ teaspoon iodized sea salt
- ¼ teaspoon crushed black pepper
- Juice of 1 lemon
- 1 teaspoon Dijon mustard
- ¼ cup extra-virgin olive oil
- 1 dash coconut aminos

Directions
- In a mixing bowl, add all of the ingredients and whisk until smooth.
- Serve immediately or refrigerate for up to a week.

Nutritional Information (per tablespoon, based on 16 servings):
- Calories: 55
- Protein: 1.2g
- Carbohydrates: 1g
- Fiber: 0.5g
- Sugar: 0g
- Fat: 5g
- Saturated Fat: 1g
- Sodium: 70mg

Vegetable Stock

NUMBER OF SERVINGS VARIES

Ingredients
- ¼ cup extra-virgin olive oil
- 2 onions, diced
- 2 parsnips, diced
- 4 celery stalks, diced
- 1 bulb fennel, chopped
- 1 cup mushrooms, chopped
- 4 cloves garlic, crushed
- 4 to 5 sprigs fresh thyme
- 1 bay leaf
- 1 small bunch parsley
- 1 teaspoon whole peppercorns
- Juice of 1 lemon
- 1 tablespoon iodized sea salt
- Enough water to cover vegetables

Directions
- Warm the olive oil in a large stockpot over medium-high heat.
- Sauté the onions, parsnips, celery, fennel, and mushrooms until they turn translucent and fragrant.
- Combine the remaining ingredients. Cover the saucepan and cook on low heat for 30 to 45 minutes.
- Strain twice and serve immediately or freeze for up to 6 months.

Nutritional Information (per 1 cup, approximately):
- Calories: 15
- Protein: 0.5g
- Carbohydrates: 2.5g
- Fiber: 0.5g
- Sugar: 1g
- Fat: 0.5g
- Saturated Fat: 0g

Lectin-Fighting Shellfish Broth

SERVES 4 TO 6

Ingredients
- 1 tablespoon extra-virgin olive oil
- 4 cups shrimp shells (from 2 pounds shrimp, fresh or frozen)
- 1 unpeeled red onion, sliced
- 2 celery stalks, sliced
- 1 bulb shallot, sliced
- 3 garlic cloves, smashed
- 1 sprig parsley
- 1 sprig thyme
- 1 sprig tarragon
- 1 to 2 bay leaves
- 1 teaspoon saffron (optional, but lovely)
- 1 teaspoon iodized sea salt
- 6 cups water, or enough to cover

Directions
- In a stockpot, warm the olive oil over medium heat. Add the shells and simmer for 10 minutes.
- Add all of the remaining ingredients, except the water.
- Increase the heat to medium-high and cook, uncovered, for 10 minutes.
- Cover and cook for another 10 minutes.
- Bring the water to a boil in the pot, then reduce heat and let it simmer for 20 minutes.
- Strain the mixture into a heatproof container.
- Use right away, or chill to room temperature before freezing for up to 6 months.

Nutritional Information (per 1 cup, approximately):
- Calories: 30
- Protein: 2g
- Carbohydrates: 2g
- Fiber: 0.5g
- Sugar: 0.5g
- Fat: 1g
- Saturated Fat: 0g

Rich Red Sauce

SERVES 4

Ingredients
- 1 tablespoon extra-virgin olive oil
- 1 medium onion, chopped finely
- 2 cloves garlic, peeled
- 1 teaspoon chopped chilli (optional)
- 1 large red capsicum, seeded and sliced

Directions
- Heat the oil in a pot, then add the onion, garlic, and chilli. Cook for 6-8 minutes, covered, over a low heat.
- Cook for an additional 10-15 minutes after adding the capsicum.
- Puree the sauce in a blender.

Nutritional Information (per serving):

- Calories: ~70
- Protein: 1.2g
- Carbohydrates: 6g
- Fiber: 1.5g
- Sugar: 3g
- Fat: 4g
- Saturated Fat: 0.5g

Cool-as-a-cucumber Sauce

SERVES 4

Ingredients

- 2 Lebanese cucumbers or 1 telegraph cucumber
- 200g natural or Greek-style yoghurt*
- 2 teaspoons finely grated lime zest
- 2 tablespoons lime juice

Directions

- Peel cucumbers, split in half, and remove the seeds.
- Dice the flesh very fine. Add the remaining ingredients.

Nutritional Information (per serving):

- Calories: ~50
- Protein: 3g
- Carbohydrates: 2g
- Fiber: 1g
- Sugar: 2g
- Fat: 2g
- Saturated Fat: 1g

Thai-style Sauce

SERVES 4

Ingredients

- ½ cup lime or lemon juice
- 1 tablespoon fish sauce
- 1 small chilli, seeded and chopped finely
- 1 stalk lemon grass, white base section, sliced very finely
- 1 tablespoon salt-reduced soy sauce
- 1 clove garlic, peeled and crushed
- ¼ cup chopped fresh mint leaves
- ½ cup chopped fresh coriander

Directions

- Combine all ingredients and leave to stand for at least 1 hour.

Nutritional Information (per serving):

- Calories: ~15
- Protein: 0.5g
- Carbohydrates: 2g
- Fiber: 1g
- Sugar: 0.5g
- Fat: 0g
- Saturated Fat: 0g

Quick Tomato Dressing

SERVES 4

Ingredients

- 500g ripe tomatoes, cores removed,

- diced finely
- ½ cup fresh basil sprigs
- ½ cup flat-leaf parsley
- freshly ground black pepper

Directions
- Place all of the ingredients in a food processor and pulse until well mixed.
- You can serve it cold or reheat it in a small saucepan.

Nutritional Information (per serving):
- Calories: ~25
- Protein: 1g
- Carbohydrates: 5g
- Fiber: 2g
- Sugar: 3g
- Fat: 0g
- Saturated Fat: 0g

Week 1 Shopping List

Vegetables
- Sweet potatoes (4 large)
- Cauliflower (1 head)
- Avocados (5 medium)
- Zucchini (4 large)
- Bell peppers (3, any color)
- Microgreens (1 small package)
- Spinach (2 cups, fresh)
- Mushrooms (1 cup, fresh)
- Asparagus (1 bunch)
- Kale (1 bunch)
- Carrots (3 medium)
- Cucumber (1 large)
- Garlic (1 bulb)
- Onions (2 large)
- Lemon (1 large)
- Mixed greens or salad greens (4 cups)
- Fresh herbs (parsley, cilantro, dill, or mint as needed)

Fruits
- Berries (blueberries, raspberries, or strawberries – 3 cups total)
- Citrus fruits (1 grapefruit or orange)
- Coconut (shredded or flakes, unsweetened)

Protein
- Eggs (14 large)
- Halibut (4 fillets or 1 pound)
- Chicken breast (2 pounds)
- Salmon (2 fillets or 1 pound)
- Moroccan-spiced chicken (1 pound or pre-seasoned)
- Shrimp (1 pound)
- Tofu (firm, 1 block)
- Turkey breast (1 pound, ground or sliced)
- Braised short ribs (1.5 pounds)
- Cod (4 fillets or 1 pound)

Grains & Legumes
- Quinoa (1 cup, dry)
- Lentils (1 cup, dry or canned)
- Millet (1/2 cup, dry)
- Miracle rice or shirataki noodles (1 package)
- Chia seeds (1/4 cup)

Dairy & Alternatives
- Plain yogurt or coconut yogurt (1 cup)
- Nutritional yeast (1/4 cup)
- Butter or ghee (optional for cooking)

Pantry Staples
- Almond flour or similar (for pancakes)
- Olive oil (for dressing and cooking)
- Pesto (1/2 cup)
- Nuts (for Dr. Gundry's mix –

- almonds, walnuts, or hazelnuts)
- Cashews (1/4 cup, raw or roasted)
- Tomato sauce (1/2 cup for spaghetti and pizza)
- Hummus (1/2 cup)
- Spices (paprika, cumin, cinnamon, turmeric, garlic powder, onion powder)
- Honey or maple syrup (optional for sweetener)

Additional Ingredients
- Cauliflower crust (pre-made or homemade)
- Microgreens (optional topping)
- Gluten-free or almond crackers

Week 1 Meal Plan

Days	Breakfast	Lunch	Snack	Dinner
Day 1	Sweet Potato Pancakes	Buffalo Cauliflower Bites	Dr. Grundy's Nut Mix	Halibut with Mushroom Ragout and Lentils
Day 2	Pesto-Baked Eggs	Chicken and Vegetable (Miracle) Rice Soup	Avocado Deviled Eggs	Sweet Potato Spaghetti and Meatballs
Day 3	Bacon-and-Egg Breakfast Salad	Grilled Salmon Salad with Citrus Dressing	Caramelized Onion Dip	Moroccan-Spiced Chicken with Millet Tabbouleh
Day 4	Chia Seed Pudding with Berries	Stuffed Bell Peppers with Lentils	Cucumber and Hummus Cups	Grilled Shrimp with Garlic Zoodles
Day 5	Spinach and Mushroom Omelet	Cauliflower Crust Veggie Pizza	Kale Chips with Nutritional Yeast	Vegetable Stir-fry with Tofu and Cashews
Day 6	Avocado Toast with Microgreens	Turkey and Avocado Lettuce Wraps	Chia Seed Crackers with Guacamole	Braised Short Ribs with Roasted Root Vegetables
Day 7	Zucchini Noodle Frittata	Mediterranean Quinoa Bowl	Berry and Coconut Yogurt Parfait	Herb-Crusted Cod with Asparagus and Quinoa

Week 2 Shopping List

Vegetables
- Zucchini (4 medium)
- Spaghetti squash (1 medium)
- Broccoli (1 head or 2 cups florets)
- Green beans (1 cup)
- Spinach (3 cups)
- Tomatoes (3 medium)
- Kale (1 bunch)
- Bok choy (2 medium heads)
- Sweet potatoes (2 medium)
- Brussels sprouts (1 pound)
- Cabbage (1 small head)
- Carrots (3 medium)
- Avocados (3 medium)
- Cauliflower (1 head or 2 cups florets)
- Garlic (1 bulb)
- Lemon (2 large)
- Fresh herbs (parsley, dill, thyme, or rosemary)

Fruits
- Mixed berries (blueberries, raspberries, strawberries – 3 cups)
- Apples (2 medium)
- Bananas (1 for smoothie bowl, optional)
- Dark chocolate (1 small bar or shavings)
- Coconut (cream or flakes, unsweetened)

Protein
- Eggs (12 large)
- Chicken breast (1.5 pounds)
- Turkey breast (1.5 pounds, ground or sliced)
- Salmon (2 fillets or 1 pound)
- Shrimp (1 pound)
- Cod (2 fillets or 1 pound)
- Tofu (1 block, firm)
- Goat cheese (1/2 cup, crumbled)

Grains & Legumes
- Almond flour (for pancakes)
- Lentils (1 cup, dry or canned)
- Chickpeas (1 cup, dry or canned)
- Wild rice (1/2 cup, dry)
- Quinoa (1 cup, dry)

Dairy & Alternatives
- Coconut yogurt (1 cup)
- Almond butter (1/2 cup)

Pantry Staples
- Olive oil (for dressing and cooking)
- Coconut oil (optional for waffles or cooking)
- Chia seeds (1/4 cup)
- Tahini (1/4 cup)
- Granola (1 cup)
- Almonds (1/4 cup, for smoothie bowl and trail mix)

- Sunflower seeds (1/4 cup, for trail mix)
- Cashews (1/4 cup, roasted or raw)
- Seaweed crisps (1 small package)
- Spices (paprika, cinnamon, turmeric, garlic powder, onion powder)

Additional Ingredients
- Gluten-free waffle mix or ingredients to make gluten-free waffles
- Vegetable broth (2 cups, for soup and curry)
- Dark chocolate shavings (optional for snacks)

Week 2 Meal Plan

Days	Breakfast	Lunch	Snack	Dinner
Day 1	Almond Flour Pancakes with Mixed Berries	Zucchini Lasagna	Roasted Spiced Chickpeas	Lemon-Herb Chicken with Steamed Broccoli
Day 2	Coconut Yogurt Parfait with Granola	Spaghetti Squash with Turkey Bolognese	Almond Butter Apple Slices	Grilled Salmon with Garlic Green Beans
Day 3	Scrambled Eggs with Spinach and Tomatoes	Kale Caesar Salad with Grilled Chicken	Veggie Sticks with Avocado Dip	Shrimp Stir-Fry with Bok Choy
Day 4	Chocolate Chia Seed Pudding	Lentil and Sweet Potato Curry	Sunflower Seed Trail Mix	Oven-Baked Cod with Roasted Brussels Sprouts
Day 5	Green Smoothie Bowl with Almonds	Cabbage and Carrot Slaw with Grilled Tofu	Seaweed Crisps with Tahini	Moroccan Chickpea Stew with Quinoa
Day 6	Poached Eggs on Avocado Toast	Wild Rice and Mushroom Soup	Roasted Cashews with Paprika	Turkey Meatballs with Zucchini Noodles
Day 7	Gluten-Free Waffles with Coconut Cream	Spinach and Goat Cheese Salad	Fresh Berry Mix with Dark Chocolate Shavings	Grilled Chicken with Roasted Cauliflower

Week 3 Shopping List

Vegetables
- Eggplants (2 medium)
- Chickpeas (1 cup, canned or cooked)
- Cauliflower (1 head or 2 cups florets)
- Bell peppers (4 medium, assorted colors)
- Zucchini (5 medium)
- Asparagus (1 bunch)
- Snap peas (1 cup)
- Kale (1 bunch)
- Spinach (2 cups, fresh)
- Mushrooms (1 cup, fresh)
- Cucumbers (2 medium)
- Sweet potatoes (2 medium)
- Avocados (3 medium)
- Celery (1 bunch)
- Garlic (1 bulb)
- Onions (2 medium)
- Fresh herbs (dill, mint, parsley, and basil as needed)

Fruits
- Bananas (2 medium)
- Apples (3 medium)
- Lemon (3 large)
- Limes (optional, for Thai curry)
- Dried fruit (e.g., raisins or cranberries for trail mix)

Protein
- Eggs (6 large)
- Chicken breast (1.5 pounds)
- Salmon (2 fillets or 1 pound)
- Shrimp (1 pound)
- Cod (2 fillets or 1 pound)
- Lamb chops (1.5 pounds)
- Tuna steaks (2 fillets or 1 pound)
- Tofu (1 block, firm)
- Feta cheese (1/2 cup, crumbled)
- Cheese for crepes (optional)

Grains & Legumes
- Oats (1 cup, for overnight oats and pancakes)
- Quinoa (1.5 cups, dry)
- Wild rice (1/2 cup, dry)
- Black beans (1 cup, canned or cooked)
- Corn (1 cup, canned or fresh)

Dairy & Alternatives
- Coconut milk (1 can, for curry and smoothie)
- Almond butter (1/4 cup)
- Peanut butter (1/4 cup)

Pantry Staples
- Olive oil (for cooking and dressing)
- Sunflower butter (1/4 cup)
- Ranch dip (or ingredients to make it)
- Hummus (1/2 cup)
- Dark chocolate (for snacks)

- Spices (cinnamon, paprika, turmeric, cumin, garlic powder)
- Matcha powder (1 tablespoon)
- Baking ingredients for zucchini bread (flour, baking powder, etc.)

Nuts & Seeds
- Walnuts (1/4 cup, for walnut butter)
- Almonds (1/2 cup, for spiced almonds and clusters)
- Trail mix ingredients (sunflower seeds, dried fruit, etc.)

Additional Ingredients
- Thai green curry paste (2 tablespoons)
- Vegetable broth (2 cups)
- Pesto (1/2 cup, for zoodles)
- Sushi rice or alternative (for sushi rolls)
- Seaweed sheets (nori, for sushi rolls)

Week 3 Meal Plan

Days	Breakfast	Lunch	Snack	Dinner
Day 1	Banana-Oat Pancakes with Walnut Butter	Grilled Eggplant and Chickpea Salad	Spicy Roasted Almonds	Herb-Roasted Chicken with Mashed Cauliflower
Day 2	Shakshuka with Bell Peppers and Feta	Quinoa-Stuffed Zucchini Boats	Celery Sticks with Sunflower Butter	Seared Salmon with Dill Sauce and Asparagus
Day 3	Matcha Smoothie with Coconut Milk	Thai Green Curry with Tofu	Mixed Veggie Chips with Hummus	Lemon Garlic Shrimp with Wild Rice
Day 4	Apple-Cinnamon Overnight Oats	Warm Lentil Salad with Roasted Vegetables	Dark Chocolate Almond Clusters	Chicken Stir-Fry with Snap Peas
Day 5	Protein Smoothie with Peanut Butter	Spinach and Quinoa Power Bowl	Sliced Bell Peppers with Ranch Dip	Baked Cod with Lemon and Kale Chips
Day 6	Zucchini Bread with Almond Butter	Cucumber and Avocado Sushi Rolls	Cinnamon-Spiced Apple Chips	Lamb Chops with Mint and Sweet Potatoes
Day 7	Savory Mushroom and Cheese Crepes	Black Bean and Corn Salad	Trail Mix with Dried Fruit	Grilled Tuna Steaks with Pesto Zoodles

Week 4 Shopping List

Vegetables
- Spinach (4 cups)
- Red cabbage (1 medium head)
- Cauliflower (1 head or 4 cups rice)
- Red bell peppers (3 medium)
- Broccoli (2 heads or 4 cups florets)
- Zucchini (3 medium)
- Sweet potatoes (2 medium)
- Tomatoes (4 medium)
- Mushrooms (1 cup, fresh)
- Green beans (1 bunch)
- Ratatouille vegetables (eggplant, zucchini, bell peppers, onion, tomatoes)
- Seaweed (for miso soup)

Fruits
- Blueberries (1 cup)
- Lemons (2 medium)
- Pears (2 medium)
- Pineapple (1 medium, fresh)
- Oranges (2 medium)
- Dates (6-8 large, for snacks)
- Apples (2 medium, for applesauce)
- Pumpkin (1 small or canned puree)

Protein
- Eggs (10 large)
- Sausage (4 links or 1/2 pound)
- Chicken breast (1 pound)
- Chicken thighs (4 pieces)
- Duck (1 medium, whole or breasts)
- Swordfish (2 fillets or 1 pound)
- Shrimp (1 pound, raw)
- Beef (1 pound, sliced for stir-fry)
- Pork chops (4 pieces or 1.5 pounds)
- Tempeh (1 block)
- Lamb (1.5 pounds)
- Tofu (1 block)

Dairy
- Yogurt (plain or Greek, 1.5 cups)
- Ricotta cheese (1/2 cup)

Grains & Legumes
- Granola (1/2 cup)
- Brown rice (1.5 cups)
- Edamame (1 cup, shelled)
- Black beans (1 cup, canned or cooked)
- Pumpkin seeds (1/2 cup)

Pantry Staples
- Olive oil (for cooking and dressing)
- Honey (1/4 cup)
- Chia seeds (1/4 cup)
- Miso paste (1 tablespoon)
- Dark chocolate (for dipping)
- Spices (pumpkin spice, cinnamon, garlic powder, paprika, etc.)

Herbs & Flavorings

- Fresh parsley (1 small bunch)
- Fresh thyme (1 small bunch)
- Fresh rosemary (1 small bunch)
- Garlic (1 bulb)

Nuts & Seeds
- Almonds (1/2 cup, for smoothie)
- Cashews (1/4 cup, for snacks)

Week 4 Meal Plan

Days	Breakfast	Lunch	Snack	Dinner
Day 1	Egg Muffins with Spinach and Sausage	Grilled Chicken Caesar Wraps	Yogurt with Honey and Granola	Roasted Duck with Red Cabbage
Day 2	Pumpkin Spice Chia Pudding	Cauliflower Rice Sushi Bowls	Edamame with Sea Salt	Grilled Swordfish with Roasted Peppers
Day 3	Blueberry Almond Smoothie	Greek Salad with Grilled Shrimp	Cashew Butter-Stuffed Dates	Beef and Broccoli Stir-Fry
Day 4	Mushroom and Herb Omelet	Ratatouille with Brown Rice	Coconut Energy Balls	Baked Chicken Thighs with Roasted Zucchini
Day 5	Lemon Ricotta Pancakes	Sweet Potato and Black Bean Tacos	Fresh Pineapple Spears	Grilled Pork Chops with Applesauce
Day 6	Avocado and Tomato Breakfast Sandwich	Miso Soup with Seaweed and Tofu	Orange Slices with Dark Chocolate Dip	Roasted Vegetable Paella
Day 7	Honey-Baked Pears with Yogurt	Grilled Tempeh and Spinach Salad	Roasted Pumpkin Seeds	Herb-Crusted Lamb with Green Beans

Conclusion

As we reach the end of *The Dr. Gundry's Diet Cookbook,* I hope you feel empowered, inspired, and excited about the possibilities that lie ahead on your journey to better health.

The recipes in this book were designed to not only nourish your body but to also support the restoration of your gut health, enhance your energy, and promote sustainable weight loss. As you've seen throughout this cookbook, the connection between what we eat and how we feel is profound. By embracing Dr. Gundry's teachings, you've taken a significant step toward optimizing your microbiome and reclaiming control over your health and well-being.

The path to healing your gut is a journey, and it's not about perfection—it's about consistency and making choices that support your long-term health. The principles outlined in this book aren't meant to be a temporary diet, but rather a sustainable lifestyle that will continue to serve you for years to come.

I encourage you to continue exploring the powerful impact that diet can have on your health. Don't be afraid to experiment with these recipes, tweak them to suit your tastes, and make them your own. Remember, the most important part of this journey is to listen to your body and trust the process.

Whether you are just starting out or have already seen the benefits of a gut-friendly, lectin-free lifestyle, know that you are on the path to healing, vitality, and optimal health. This book is just one piece of the puzzle, and the more you incorporate these practices into your life, the greater the transformation you'll experience.

Thank you for allowing me to be a part of your journey. I wish you the best of health, happiness, and a vibrant future.

To your continued success in health and healing,
Sonia Jones

Printed in Great Britain
by Amazon